BODY WEALTH

KITCHEN

The Balanced Plate Recipe Cookbook

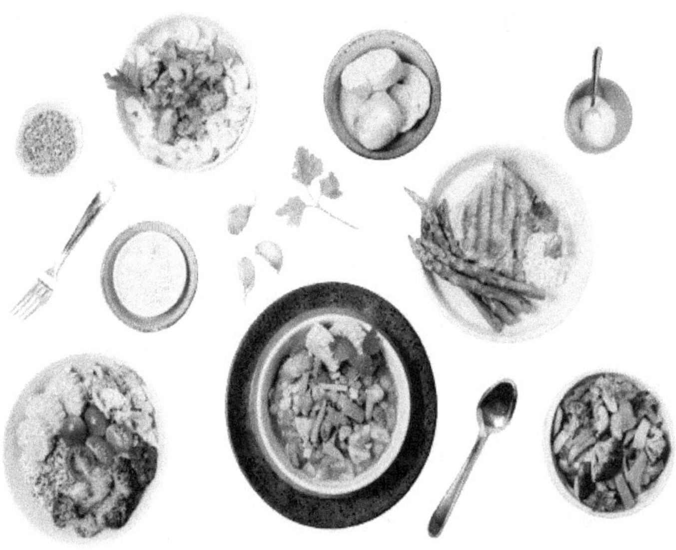

AULYN BILL

CONTENTS

PREFACE

Welcome to Healthy Eating Recipes Cookbook! This cookbook helps you reach your health and wellness goals by providing delicious and nutritious food recipes, meal planning strategies, and tips for grocery shopping and meal preparation. is designed to achieve

Eating a healthy diet is essential to maintaining optimal health and wellness, but knowing where to start can be difficult. By providing meals, we aim to make nutritious meals more accessible and enjoyable.

In this cookbook, you'll find recipes for a variety of healthy meals designed to support your health and wellness goals. Each recipe contains the macronutrients and micronutrients your body needs to thrive. Packed with nutrient-dense ingredients that provide nutrients. In addition to recipes, this cookbook also includes information on macro and micronutrients, meal planning strategies, and tips for grocery shopping and meal prep. By applying the tips, you can make healthy eating more manageable and part of your daily routine.

Whether you want to lose weight, improve your energy levels, or get in better shape, this cookbook is a valuable resource for anyone trying to adopt a healthier lifestyle. So let's nourish your body with delicious and nutritious meals and start cooking!

INTRODUCTION

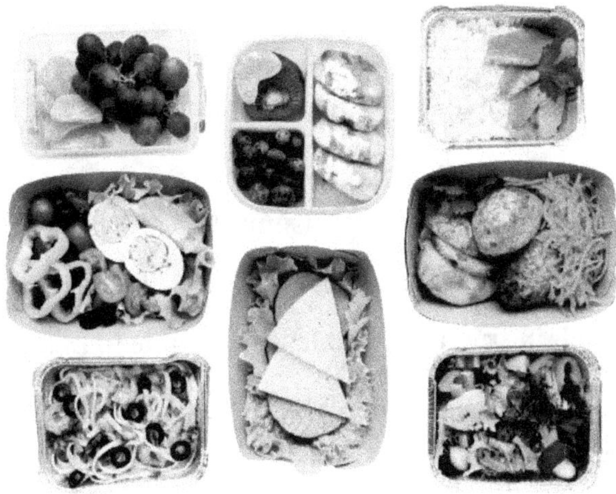

Consuming nutritious meals is crucial for maintaining excellent health and preventing persistent ailments. A well-balanced and healthy diet can supply the body with the essential vitamins, minerals, and nutrients to function effectively. It can also help maintain a healthy weight and decrease the likelihood of heart disease, stroke, diabetes, and specific cancers. It refreshes the body and serves as an anti-ageing.

Healthy eating patterns begin with integrating an array of nutrient-rich foods into your diet, such as whole grains, lean proteins, fruits, vegetables, and healthy fats. Refraining from processed and high-calorie foods can assist you in managing your weight and enhancing your overall health.

Apart from physical health, consuming healthy meals can also have a positive impact on mental health. Research has shown that a diet rich in fruits, vegetables, and whole grains can elevate mood, and cognitive function, and reduce symptoms of depression and anxiety.

Making healthy food choices can be challenging, but it is an investment in your long-term health and well-being. With the right resources and knowledge, you can create a balanced and enjoyable diet that promotes a healthy lifestyle.

Cooking your meals at home provides numerous benefits beyond just nourishing your body. Preparing your meals from scratch can be a creative and fulfilling experience that enables you to experiment with new ingredients, flavors, and cooking techniques. Here are some of the significant benefits of cooking your meals:

Regulating ingredients, conserving money, promoting healthy eating, bonding with family and friends, and reducing food waste.

This recipe book is intended to help you attain a healthy lifestyle by offering a broad range of delicious and nutritious meal options. The recipes are meticulously selected to ensure that they are balanced and brimming with healthy ingredients that provide your body with the nutrients it requires to thrive.

Whether you are a seasoned cook or a novice, this cookbook caters to everyone. The recipes are simple to follow, and each one includes a list of ingredients, step-by-step instructions, and nutritional information to help you make informed decisions about what you eat.

In addition to the recipes, this cookbook contains meal planning strategies, grocery shopping and food prep tips, and guidance on how to integrate healthy eating habits into your daily routine.

You will also find recommendations for healthy snacks, appetizers, and desserts that will satiate your cravings without compromising your health goals.

By utilizing this cookbook, you will be able to take charge of your diet and make healthier food choices that promote long-term health and wellness. Whether you are aiming to lose weight, reduce your risk of chronic disease, or simply feel better

CHAPTER 1

UNDERSTANDING HEALTHY DIET

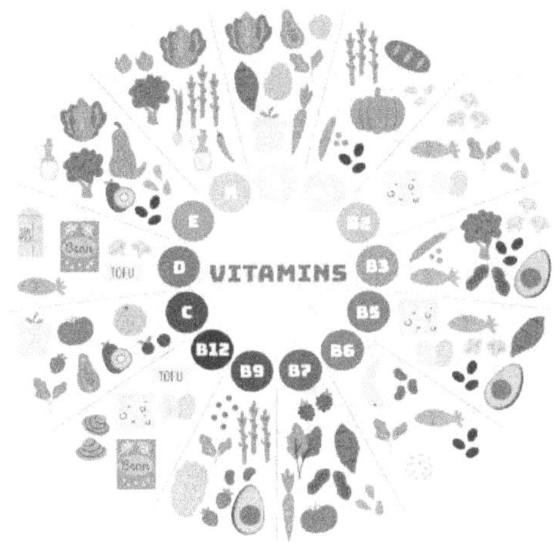

Essential diet nutrients needed

An optimal state of health and well-being requires a balanced diet rich in nutrient-packed foods. To achieve this, we must consume a diverse range of essential nutrients, including:

Protein: This macronutrient is vital for repairing and building tissues, as well as maintaining muscle mass. Excellent protein sources include lean meats, fish, poultry, eggs, legumes, and tofu.

Carbohydrates: Carbs are the body's primary energy source. They come in two forms: complex carbohydrates found in whole grains, fruits, and vegetables, and simple carbohydrates found in sugar and refined grains.

Healthy fats: Good fats provide energy and support cell growth. They can be found in nuts, seeds, avocados, fatty fish, and olive oil.

Vitamins: These micronutrients are necessary for the body to function correctly. Each vitamin has a unique function, and it can be found in fruits, vegetables, whole grains, and fortified foods.

Minerals: These micronutrients are also essential for many bodily functions, including bone health, muscle function, and nerve function. Dairy products, leafy greens, nuts, and whole grains are excellent sources of minerals.

Fiber: This nutrient is essential for digestive health and can help regulate blood sugar levels and lower cholesterol. Fruits, vegetables, whole grains, legumes, and nuts are all great sources of fiber.

Portion control and balancing food

Maintaining a healthy diet requires paying attention to portion sizes and ensuring a balance of food groups. The following explains why this is important:

Portion management: Consuming excessive quantities of any type of food can result in weight gain and other health issues. Portion control necessitates eating the right amount of food for your specific requirements. You may accomplish this by using measuring cups, a food scale, or other portion control tools. Additionally, it is critical to pay attention to your body and cease eating when you feel full.

Food group balance: A well-balanced diet that includes all food groups is essential for obtaining all of the essential nutrients your body requires. A balanced diet should include:

Fruits and vegetables: These are abundant in vitamins, minerals, and fiber.

Whole grains: These provide energy and are an excellent source of fiber.

Lean proteins: These are crucial for building and repairing tissues in the body.

Healthy fats: These provide energy and support cell growth.

By balancing these food groups, you can ensure that you are obtaining all of the essential nutrients your body requires to function correctly.

Food labels and informed choices

Acquiring the ability to read food labels is a crucial skill for making informed decisions about your diet. The following are some recommendations for interpreting food labels:

Review the serving size: The serving size is the quantity of food that the label is based on. Ensure that you check the serving size to guarantee that you are comparing similar products.

Examine the calorie count: The number of calories per serving is listed on the label. This can help you keep track of your calorie consumption.

Inspect the ingredients: The ingredients list discloses what is in the food. Ingredients are arranged in descending order of weight, so the first ingredient is the most abundant. Look for foods with whole, minimally processed ingredients.

Evaluate the nutrients: The label will specify the quantity of different nutrients in the food. Look for foods that are rich in fiber, vitamins, and minerals, and low in saturated and trans fats, added sugars, and sodium.

Utilize the % Daily Value: The % Daily Value (%DV) informs you how much of a nutrient is in a serving of food relative to the daily recommended amount. Use the %DV to compare different products and choose ones that are higher in nutrients and lower in unhealthy ingredients.

CHAPTER 2

HEALTHY DIET EATING

Tips for diabetes, heart disease, high blood pressure, cancer, overweight and other conditions

Listed below are some general guidelines for maintaining a healthy diet if you have diabetes, heart disease, high blood pressure, or other ailments:

Emphasize whole, unrefined foods: These are foods that are either minimally processed or not processed at all. For instance, fruits, vegetables, whole grains, lean proteins, and healthy fats are all examples. These foods are abundant in essential nutrients and are usually low in added sugars, sodium, and unhealthy fats.

Restrict sodium consumption: Consuming an excessive amount of sodium can raise blood pressure, which is a risk factor for heart disease and stroke. Instead of salt, use herbs and spices when cooking, read food labels for sodium content, and avoid processed foods, which are typically high in sodium.

Choose healthy fats: Healthy fats, such as those found in nuts, seeds, avocados, and fatty fish, can help lower cholesterol levels and reduce the risk of heart disease. Avoid saturated and trans fats, which can raise cholesterol levels and contribute to heart disease.

Consume a variety of fruits and vegetables: Various fruits and vegetables contain diverse vitamins, minerals, and antioxidants, so it's crucial to consume a range of them. Strive for at least five servings of fruits and vegetables per day.

Select complex carbohydrates: Complex carbohydrates, such as those found in whole grains, legumes, and starchy vegetables, provide a gradual and stable energy release and can help control blood sugar levels. Simple carbohydrates, such as those found in sugary drinks and snacks, should be avoided since they can cause blood sugar levels to spike.

Monitor your portion sizes: Even healthy foods can lead to weight gain and other health issues if eaten in large amounts. Use portion control to keep your calorie intake in check.

By adhering to these recommendations, you can maintain a healthy diet that supports your medical condition and overall health.

Foods to avoid and alternatives

When it comes to adhering to a nourishing diet for health conditions such as diabetes, heart disease or hypertension, it's crucial to concentrate on not only the foods to incorporate but also the foods to evade. Here are some foods to restrict or eliminate, as well as suggested substitutes:

Sweetened beverages: Sweetened beverages like soda, fruit juice, and sweetened tea or coffee can have a high amount of added sugars and calories. Instead, opt for water, unsweetened tea or coffee, or low-calorie alternatives such as seltzer water with a hint of fruit juice.

Processed meats: Processed meats such as bacon, sausage, and deli meats can contain an excessive amount of sodium, unhealthy fats, and additives. Instead, go for lean proteins like chicken, fish, or legumes.

Fried foods: Fried foods such as french fries, fried chicken, and fried fish can have an abundant amount of unhealthy fats and calories. Instead, experiment with baking, grilling, or roasting your preferred foods for a healthier alternative.

Refined bread and pasta: Refined bread and pasta can be high in simple carbohydrates and low in fiber. Instead, choose whole-grain bread and pasta, which have more fiber and can help regulate blood sugar levels.

High-fat dairy products: High-fat dairy products like whole milk, cheese, and cream can contain a high amount of saturated fat. Instead, select low-fat or non-fat dairy products such as skim milk, low-fat cheese, or non-fat yogurt.

By making these uncomplicated substitutions, you can still relish delicious and gratifying meals while also supporting your health and medical condition. As always, it's essential to collaborate with a healthcare professional or registered dietitian to determine the most suitable dietary approach for your individual requirements.

Meal planning strategies

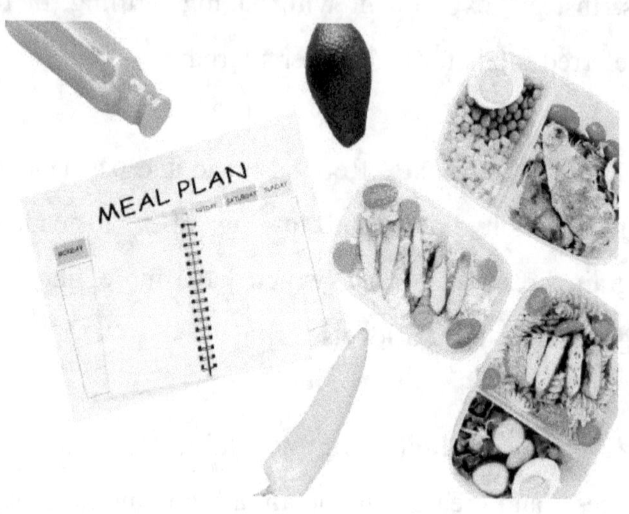

Planning your meals is an essential aspect of maintaining a healthy diet and can aid in time and money management while ensuring a well-balanced and nutritious diet. Here are some tactics for meal planning that can help you attain your health and wellness objectives:

Establish a routine: Dedicate a specific time each week to plan your meals and snacks. This could be on a weekend afternoon or any other day that suits you.

Create a grocery list: Once you have your meal plans in place, create a shopping list of the ingredients you will require. This will prevent impulsive purchases and ensure that you have everything necessary to prepare your meals.

Cook in batches: Batch cooking is a fantastic method to save time and ensure that you always have healthy meals ready to eat. Reserve a few hours each week to cook large batches of food that you can store in the fridge or freezer for later consumption.

Mix and match: Adopt a mix-and-match approach to meal planning, where you prepare various ingredients that can be combined in different ways to create diverse meals throughout the week.

Consider your schedule: When planning your meals, take into account your schedule and plan accordingly. If you know that you will be busy on particular days, prepare meals that are quick and easy to make.

Utilize leftovers: Leftovers can be an excellent way to minimize food waste and save time in the kitchen. Plan to cook extra portions of your meals and use the leftovers for lunches or dinners later in the week.

By following these meal planning techniques, you can make healthy eating a regular part of your daily routine and pave the way for success in achieving your health and wellness objectives.

Tips for grocery shopping and food prep

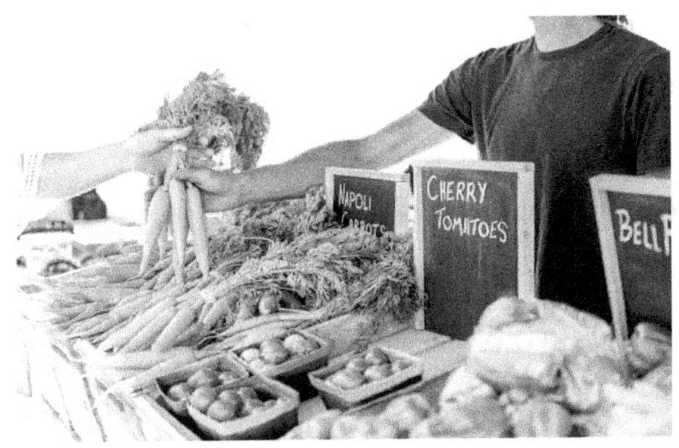

Healthy eating requires grocery shopping and food preparation, and there are some tips and techniques that can make the process more convenient and effective. Here are some suggestions for grocery shopping and food preparation:

Create a checklist: Prior to going to the supermarket, prepare a checklist of the ingredients needed for your meals. This will help you avoid unplanned purchases and ensure that you have all the necessary items for healthy meals.

Shop the outer edges: The outer edges of the grocery store typically have fresh fruits, meats, and dairy products, which are all vital elements of a healthy diet. Try to avoid the processed and packaged foods in the middle aisles of the store.

Purchase in large quantities: Purchasing in large quantities can help you save money and reduce packaging waste. Consider purchasing bulk items such as grains, beans, and nuts to use in your meals.

Prepare in advance: Preparing ingredients in advance can help you save time during the week. Cut vegetables, cook grains, and prepare snacks ahead of time so that you have healthy options readily available when you need them.

Utilize convenience products: Convenience items such as pre-cut vegetables, canned beans, and frozen fruits and vegetables can save time and make healthy eating more accessible.

Invest in high-quality tools: Investing in high-quality kitchen tools such as sharp knives, a food processor, and a blender can make food preparation easier and more efficient.

CHAPTER 3

33 VARIETY DIET RECIPES

Grilled chicken breast with roasted vegetables

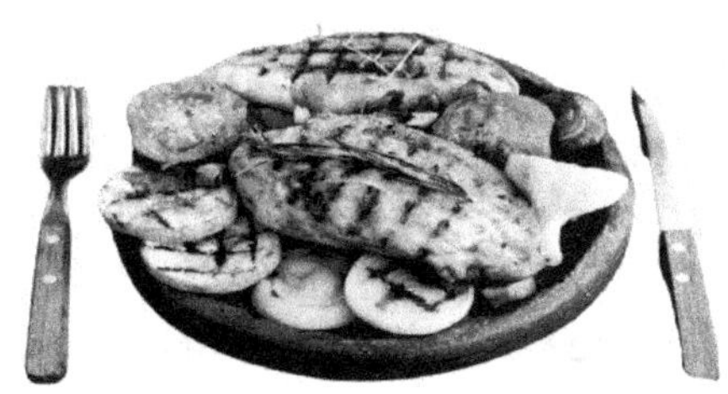

Ingredients:

2 chicken breasts

2 cups of mixed vegetables (such as broccoli, bell peppers, onions, and zucchini)

2 tablespoons of olive oil

1 teaspoon of salt

1/2 teaspoon of black pepper

1 teaspoon of garlic powder

1 teaspoon of dried oregano

Instructions:

- Preheat the oven to 400°F (200°C).
- Cut the vegetables into bite-sized pieces and place them in a large mixing bowl.
- Add 1 tablespoon of olive oil, 1/2 teaspoon of salt, and 1/4 teaspoon of black pepper to the vegetables. Toss to coat the vegetables evenly with the oil and seasoning.
- Spread the vegetables evenly onto a baking sheet and roast them in the oven for 20-25 minutes or until they are tender and lightly browned.
- While the vegetables are roasting, season the chicken breasts with 1/2 teaspoon of salt, 1/4 teaspoon of black pepper, 1 teaspoon of garlic powder, and 1 teaspoon of dried oregano.
- Heat a grill pan or outdoor grill over medium-high heat. Brush the chicken breasts with 1 tablespoon of olive oil.
- Grill the chicken breasts for 6-8 minutes on each side or until they are cooked through and no longer pink in the center.

Serve the grilled chicken breasts with the roasted vegetables.

Baked salmon with quinoa and sautéed spinach

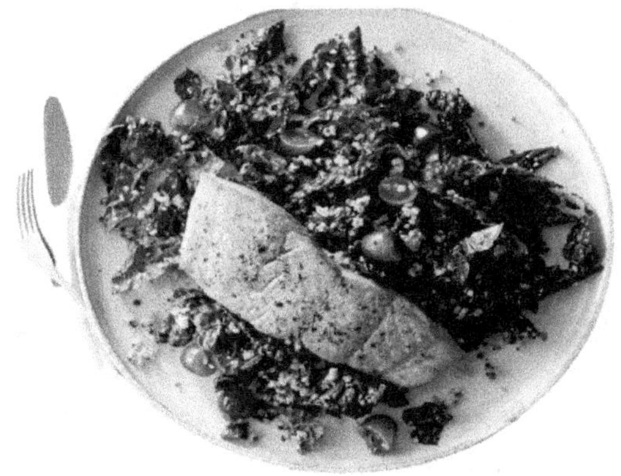

Ingredients:

4 salmon fillets (about 6 ounces each)

1 cup of quinoa

2 cups of water

2 tablespoons of olive oil, divided

1 teaspoon of salt, divided

1/2 teaspoon of black pepper, divided

1 teaspoon of garlic powder

1 teaspoon of paprika

8 cups of fresh spinach

Instructions:

- Preheat the oven to 375°F (190°C).

- Rinse the quinoa thoroughly and add it to a medium-sized saucepan with 2 cups of water and 1/2 teaspoon of salt. Bring to a boil, then reduce heat to low and simmer for 18-20 minutes, or until the quinoa is tender and the water has been absorbed.

- Season the salmon fillets with 1/2 teaspoon of salt, 1/4 teaspoon of black pepper, 1 teaspoon of garlic powder, and 1 teaspoon of paprika.

- Heat 1 tablespoon of olive oil in a large skillet over medium heat. Add the spinach and sauté for 2-3 minutes or until wilted. Season with 1/4 teaspoon of salt and 1/4 teaspoon of black pepper.

- Heat 1 tablespoon of olive oil in another large oven-safe skillet over medium-high heat. Add the salmon fillets and cook for 3-4 minutes on each side until browned. Transfer the skillet to the preheated oven and bake for an additional 8-10 minutes, or until the salmon is cooked through and flakes easily with a fork.

Serve the salmon fillets with the cooked quinoa and sautéed spinach.

Lentil soup with whole-grain bread

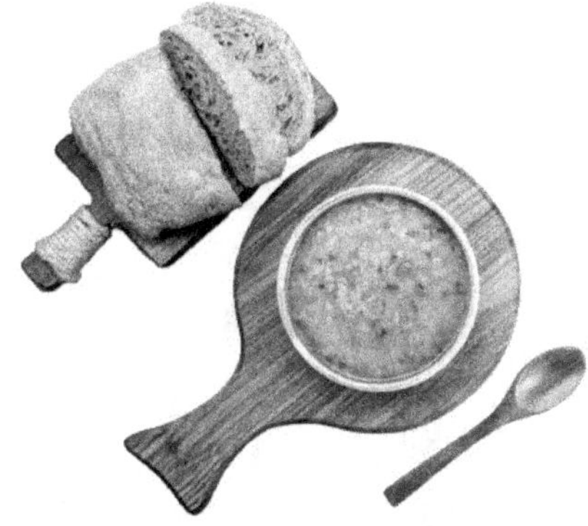

Ingredients:

For the lentil soup:

1 cup of dry brown or green lentils

1 onion, diced

2 garlic cloves, minced

2 celery stalks, chopped

2 carrots, chopped

1 teaspoon of ground cumin

1 teaspoon of smoked paprika

4 cups of vegetable broth

1 cup of water

1 tablespoon of olive oil

Salt and pepper to taste

Fresh parsley or cilantro, chopped (optional)

For the whole grain bread:

2 cups of whole wheat flour

1 cup of all-purpose flour

1 tablespoon of honey

2 teaspoons of active dry yeast

1 teaspoon of salt

1 1/4 cups of warm water

Instructions:

For the lentil soup:

- Rinse the lentils in a strainer and set aside.
- In a large pot, heat the olive oil over medium heat. Add the onions, garlic, celery, and carrots and cook until the vegetables are tender about 5-7 minutes.

- Add the ground cumin and smoked paprika and cook for an additional minute, stirring frequently.
- Add the lentils, vegetable broth, and water to the pot. Bring to a boil, then reduce the heat to low and simmer for 30-40 minutes or until the lentils are tender.
- Season the soup with salt and pepper to taste.

If desired, garnish with fresh parsley or cilantro.

For the whole grain bread:

- In a large mixing bowl, combine the whole wheat flour, all-purpose flour, honey, yeast, and salt.
- Slowly add the warm water while mixing until the dough comes together and forms a ball.
- Knead the dough for 10 minutes on a lightly floured surface until it becomes smooth and elastic.
- Place the dough in a greased bowl, cover it with a cloth, and let it rise in a warm place for 1 hour or until it has doubled in size.
- Preheat the oven to 375°F (190°C).
- Punch down the dough and shape it into a loaf. Place the loaf in a greased bread pan and let it rise for an additional 30 minutes.

- Bake the bread for 35-40 minutes or until it is golden brown and sounds hollow when tapped.

Let the bread cool before slicing.

Grilled tofu with brown rice and steamed broccoli

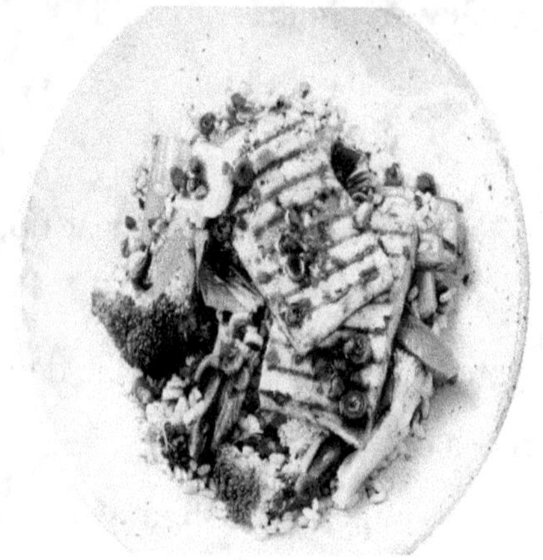

Ingredients:

For the grilled tofu:

1 block of firm or extra-firm tofu, drained and pressed

1/4 cup of soy sauce

2 tablespoons of maple syrup

1 tablespoon of rice vinegar

1 tablespoon of sesame oil

1 teaspoon of grated ginger

2 garlic cloves, minced

For the brown rice:

1 cup of brown rice

2 cups of water

Salt to taste

For the steamed broccoli:

1 head of broccoli, cut into florets

Water for steaming

Instructions:

For the grilled tofu:

- Cut the pressed tofu into slices or cubes.
- In a mixing bowl, whisk together the soy sauce, maple syrup, rice vinegar, sesame oil, grated ginger, and minced garlic.
- Add the tofu to the mixing bowl and toss to coat evenly. Let marinate for at least 30 minutes, or up to overnight.

- Heat a grill or grill pan over medium-high heat. Grill the tofu for 5-7 minutes on each side, or until grill marks appear.

For the brown rice:

- Rinse the brown rice in a fine-mesh strainer and drain.
- In a medium pot, combine the rice, water, and salt. Bring to a boil over high heat, then reduce the heat to low and cover the pot with a tight-fitting lid.
- Simmer the rice for 40-45 minutes, or until the water has been absorbed and the rice is tender.

For the steamed broccoli:

- Bring a pot of water to a boil.
- Place the broccoli florets in a steamer basket and set it over the pot of boiling water.
- Cover the pot with a lid and steam the broccoli for 3-4 minutes, or until it is bright green and tender.

Serve the grilled tofu with brown rice and steamed broccoli.

Grilled shrimp with stir-fried vegetables and brown rice noodles

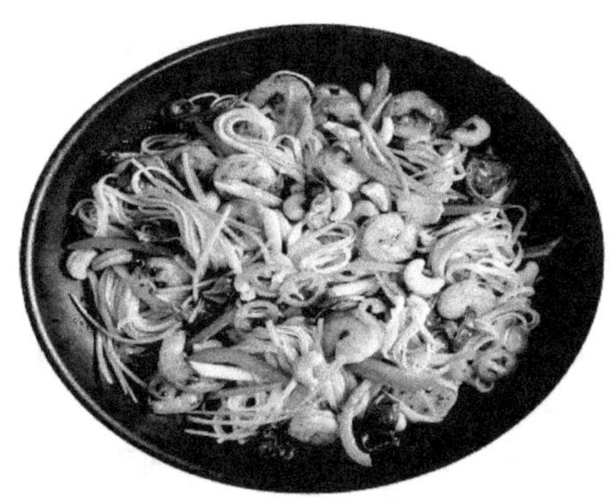

Ingredients:

For the grilled shrimp:

1 lb. of large shrimp, peeled and deveined

1 tablespoon of olive oil

1 teaspoon of paprika

1 teaspoon of garlic powder

Salt and pepper to taste

For the stir-fried vegetables:

1 red bell pepper, sliced

1 yellow bell pepper, sliced

1 small onion, sliced

1 cup of sliced mushrooms

2 cloves of garlic, minced

1 tablespoon of olive oil

Salt and pepper to taste

For the brown rice noodles:

8 oz. of brown rice noodles

Water for boiling

Salt to taste

For the sauce:

2 tablespoons of soy sauce

2 tablespoons of honey

1 tablespoon of rice vinegar

1 tablespoon of sesame oil

1 tablespoon of cornstarch

1/4 cup of water

Instructions:

- In a mixing bowl, toss the peeled and deveined shrimp with olive oil, paprika, garlic powder, salt, and pepper.
- Heat a grill or grill pan over medium-high heat.
- Grill the shrimp for 2-3 minutes on each side, or until they are pink and cooked through.

- Heat a wok or large skillet over high heat.
- Add olive oil and swirl to coat the pan.
- Add the sliced bell peppers, onion, mushrooms, garlic, salt, and pepper to the pan and stir-fry for 3-4 minutes, or until the vegetables are tender-crisp.

- Bring a pot of salted water to a boil.
- Add the brown rice noodles to the boiling water and cook for 4-6 minutes, or until they are tender.
- Drain the noodles and rinse them with cold water to stop the cooking process.

For the sauce:

- In a small bowl, whisk together the soy sauce, honey, rice vinegar, sesame oil, cornstarch, and water.

Set aside.

To assemble the dish:

- Arrange the cooked shrimp on a serving plate.
- In a mixing bowl, toss the cooked brown rice noodles with the stir-fried vegetables.
- Pour the sauce over the noodles and vegetables and toss to coat evenly.
- Serve the noodles and vegetables alongside the grilled shrimp.

Greek yogurt with mixed berries and granola

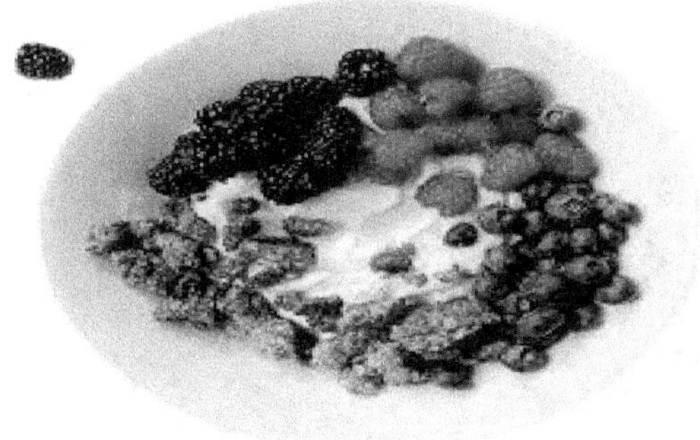

Ingredients:

1 cup of plain Greek yogurt

1 cup of mixed berries (such as strawberries, blueberries, and raspberries)

1/4 cup of granola

Instructions:

- Rinse the mixed berries under cold water and pat them dry with a paper towel.
- In a small mixing bowl, mix together the Greek yogurt and mixed berries.
- Sprinkle the granola on top of the yogurt and berries.

Serve immediately.

Avocado toast with poached egg and sliced tomato

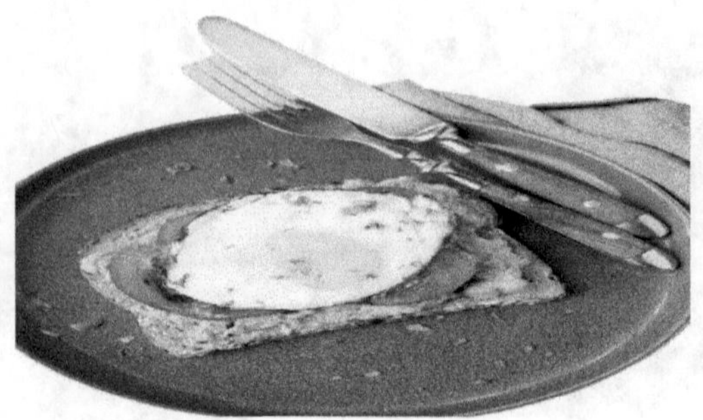

Ingredients:

2 slices of whole-grain bread

1 ripe avocado

1 medium-sized tomato, sliced

2 large eggs

1 tablespoon of white vinegar

Salt and pepper to taste

Instructions:

- Toast the slices of whole-grain bread until they are golden brown.
- Cut the avocado in half and remove the pit. Scoop out the flesh into a bowl and mash it with a fork.

- Spread the mashed avocado evenly onto the slices of toasted bread.

- Top the avocado toast with sliced tomato.

- Bring a pot of water to a simmer over medium-high heat. Add white vinegar to the pot.

- Crack one egg into a small bowl. Using a slotted spoon, create a whirlpool in the simmering water, then slide the egg into the water.

- Poach the egg for 2-3 minutes, or until the whites are set and the yolks are still runny.

- Use the slotted spoon to remove the poached egg from the water and place it on top of the sliced tomato on one of the pieces of toast.

Repeat steps 6-8 with the second egg.

- Season the poached eggs with salt and pepper to taste.

Serve immediately.

Black bean and vegetable stir-fry with brown rice

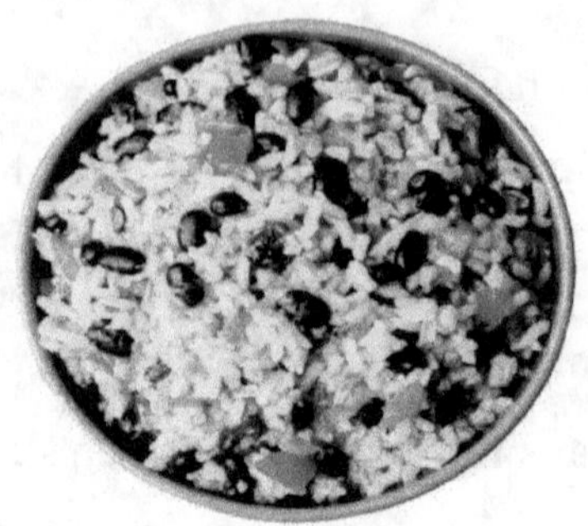

Ingredients:

1 cup of brown rice

1 tablespoon of vegetable oil

1 onion, chopped

2 garlic cloves, minced

1 red bell pepper, chopped

1 zucchini, chopped

1 cup of sliced mushrooms

1 can (15 ounces) of black beans, drained and rinsed

1 tablespoon of low-sodium soy sauce

1 teaspoon of ground cumin

1/4 teaspoon of chili powder

Salt and pepper to taste

Instructions:

- Cook the brown rice according to package instructions and set aside.
- In a large wok or frying pan, heat the vegetable oil over medium-high heat.
- Add the chopped onion and minced garlic and stir-fry for 2-3 minutes, or until the onion is translucent.
- Add the chopped red bell pepper, zucchini, and sliced mushrooms to the pan and stir-fry for another 5-7 minutes, or until the vegetables are tender.
- Add the drained and rinsed black beans, soy sauce, ground cumin, and chili powder to the pan and stir-fry for another 2-3 minutes, or until the beans are heated through.
- Season the stir-fry with salt and pepper to taste.

Serve the black bean and vegetable stir-fry over the cooked brown rice.

Roasted sweet potato and black bean tacos

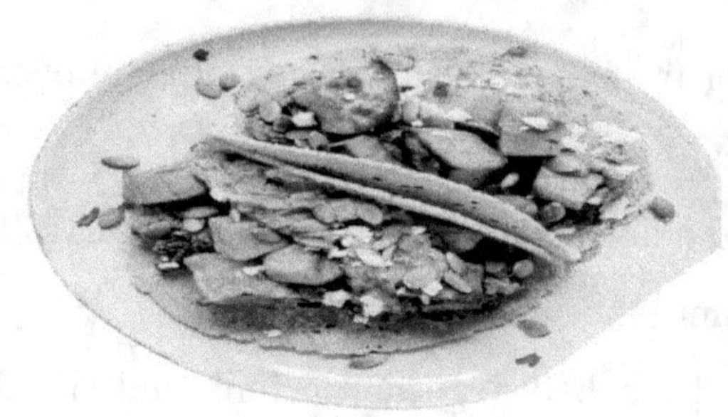

Ingredients:

2 medium-sized sweet potatoes, peeled and diced

1 tablespoon of olive oil

1 teaspoon of chili powder

1/2 teaspoon of ground cumin

Salt and pepper to taste

1 can (15 ounces) of black beans, drained and rinsed

1 small red onion, diced

1/4 cup of chopped fresh cilantro

Juice of 1 lime

8 small tortillas

Optional toppings: sliced avocado, salsa, shredded cheese, sour cream

Instructions:

- Preheat the oven to 400°F (200°C).

- In a large bowl, toss the diced sweet potatoes with olive oil, chili powder, cumin, salt, and pepper.

- Spread the seasoned sweet potatoes in a single layer on a baking sheet and roast in the preheated oven for 20-25 minutes, or until they are tender and lightly browned.

- In a small bowl, mix the drained and rinsed black beans with diced red onion, chopped cilantro, and lime juice.

Warm the tortillas in a pan or in the microwave.

- Assemble the tacos by filling each tortilla with roasted sweet potatoes and black bean mixture.

- Add optional toppings as desired.

Serve immediately.

Chicken and vegetable stir-fry with quinoa

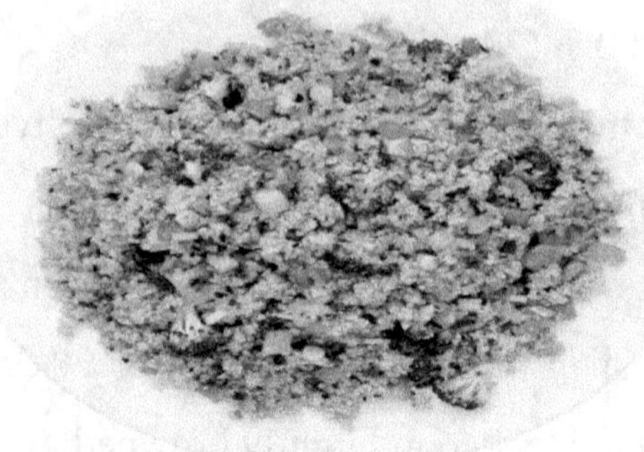

Ingredients:

1 cup of quinoa

2 cups of water

1 tablespoon of vegetable oil

1 pound of boneless, skinless chicken breasts, cut into small pieces

Salt and pepper to taste

2 cloves of garlic, minced

1 red bell pepper, sliced

1 zucchini, sliced

1 cup of sliced mushrooms

2 tablespoons of low-sodium soy sauce

1 tablespoon of honey

1 teaspoon of grated fresh ginger

1/4 teaspoon of red pepper flakes (optional)

Instructions:

- Rinse the quinoa thoroughly and add it to a medium saucepan with 2 cups of water. Bring to a boil, reduce heat to low, cover and simmer for 15-20 minutes, or until the quinoa is cooked and the water is absorbed.
- In a large wok or frying pan, heat the vegetable oil over medium-high heat.
- Season the chicken pieces with salt and pepper and add them to the pan. Stir-fry for 5-7 minutes, or until the chicken is cooked through and lightly browned.
- Add the minced garlic, sliced red bell pepper, sliced zucchini, and sliced mushrooms to the pan and stir-fry for another 5-7 minutes, or until the vegetables are tender.
- In a small bowl, whisk together the low-sodium soy sauce, honey, grated fresh ginger, and red pepper flakes (if using).
- Pour the sauce over the chicken and vegetables and stir-fry for another 2-3 minutes, or until the sauce is

heated through and the chicken and vegetables are evenly coated.

Serve the chicken and vegetable stir-fry over the cooked quinoa.

Grilled steak with roasted sweet potato and green beans

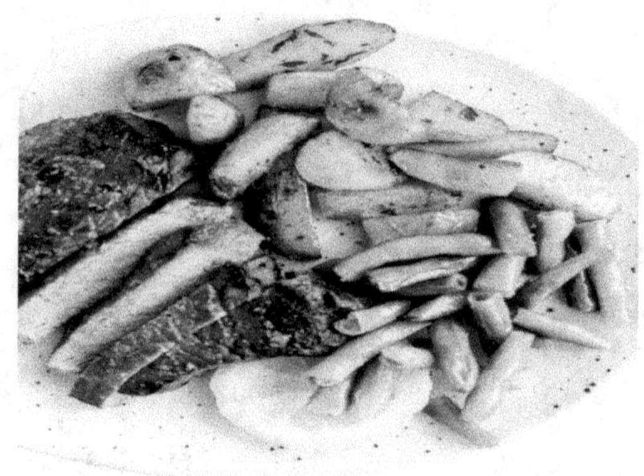

Ingredients:

1 pound of sirloin steak

1 tablespoon of olive oil

Salt and pepper to taste

2 medium sweet potatoes, peeled and chopped into bite-sized pieces

1 pound of fresh green beans, trimmed

1 tablespoon of balsamic vinegar

1 tablespoon of honey

1 tablespoon of Dijon mustard

Instructions:

- Preheat the oven to 425°F.
- Rub the steak with olive oil and season it with salt and pepper.
- Grill the steak on medium-high heat for 4-5 minutes per side for medium-rare, or until it reaches your desired level of doneness.
- Let the steak rest for 5-10 minutes before slicing it thinly against the grain.
- While the steak is cooking, toss the chopped sweet potatoes with 1 tablespoon of olive oil and salt and pepper to taste.
- Spread them out in a single layer on a baking sheet and roast in the preheated oven for 25-30 minutes, or until they are tender and lightly browned.
- Toss the trimmed green beans with 1 tablespoon of olive oil and salt and pepper to taste. Spread them out in a

single layer on a separate baking sheet and roast in the preheated oven for 12-15 minutes, or until they are tender and lightly browned.

- In a small bowl, whisk together the balsamic vinegar, honey, and Dijon mustard to make a sauce.

Serve the sliced steak with the roasted sweet potatoes and green beans, and drizzle the sauce over the top.

Grilled portobello mushrooms with mixed greens and balsamic vinaigrette

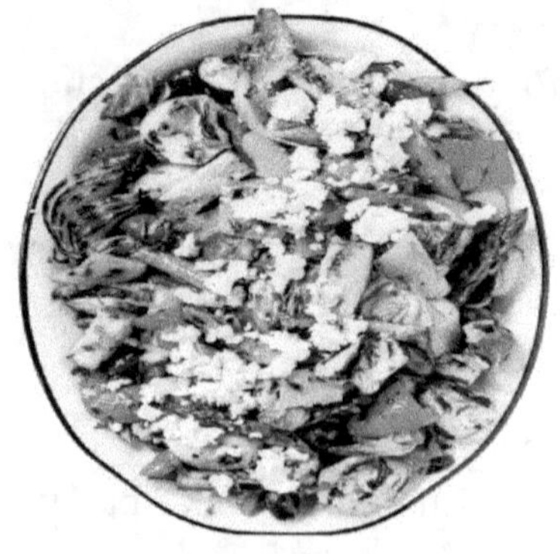

Ingredients:

4 large portobello mushroom caps

2 tablespoons of olive oil

Salt and pepper to taste

6 cups of mixed greens

1/2 cup of cherry tomatoes, halved

1/4 cup of crumbled feta cheese

1/4 cup of chopped walnuts

3 tablespoons of balsamic vinegar

2 tablespoons of olive oil

1 teaspoon of Dijon mustard

1 teaspoon of honey

Salt and pepper to taste

Instructions:

- Preheat the grill to medium-high heat.
- Brush the portobello mushroom caps with olive oil and season them with salt and pepper.
- Grill the mushrooms for 4-5 minutes per side, or until they are tender and lightly charred.
- While the mushrooms are cooking, prepare the mixed greens by tossing them with cherry tomatoes, crumbled feta cheese, and chopped walnuts in a large bowl.

- In a small bowl, whisk together the balsamic vinegar, olive oil, Dijon mustard, honey, salt, and pepper to make a dressing.
- Drizzle the dressing over the mixed greens and toss to combine.

Serve the grilled portobello mushrooms alongside the mixed greens salad.

Turkey chili with mixed vegetables and quinoa

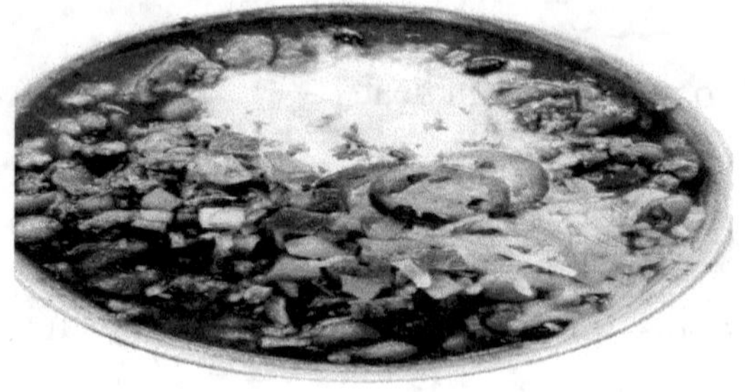

Ingredients:

1 pound ground turkey

1 tablespoon olive oil

1 onion, chopped

3 cloves garlic, minced

1 red bell pepper, chopped

1 green bell pepper, chopped

1 can (15 ounces) diced tomatoes

1 can (15 ounces) kidney beans, drained and rinsed

1 can (15 ounces) black beans, drained and rinsed

1 cup frozen corn

1 cup uncooked quinoa, rinsed

1 tablespoon chili powder

1 teaspoon cumin

1 teaspoon smoked paprika

Salt and pepper to taste

4 cups low-sodium chicken broth

Optional toppings: shredded cheese, chopped green onions, sour cream

Instructions:

- Heat the olive oil in a large pot or Dutch oven over medium-high heat.
- Add the ground turkey, onion, garlic, and bell peppers. Cook, stirring occasionally, until the turkey is browned and the vegetables are tender.

- Add the diced tomatoes, kidney beans, black beans, corn, quinoa, chili powder, cumin, smoked paprika, salt, and pepper. Stir to combine.
- Pour in the chicken broth and bring the mixture to a boil.
- Reduce the heat to medium-low and simmer the chili for 25-30 minutes, or until the quinoa is tender and the flavors have melded together.

Serve the chili hot, topped with shredded cheese, chopped green onions, and/or sour cream, if desired.

Grilled salmon with roasted asparagus and sweet potato fries

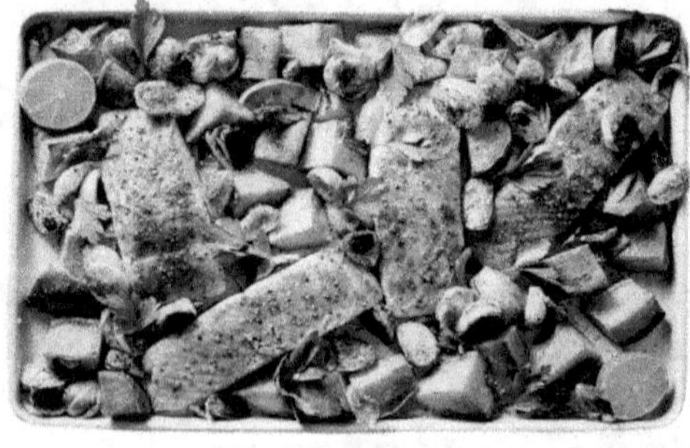

Ingredients:

4 salmon fillets

1 tablespoon olive oil

Salt and pepper to taste

1 bunch asparagus, trimmed

2 large sweet potatoes, cut into fries

1 tablespoon cornstarch

1 teaspoon smoked paprika

1/2 teaspoon garlic powder

Optional toppings: lemon wedges, chopped parsley

Instructions:

- Preheat the oven to 425°F (218°C). Line a baking sheet with parchment paper.
- Toss the sweet potato fries with the cornstarch, smoked paprika, garlic powder, salt, and pepper until coated.
- Arrange the sweet potato fries in a single layer on the prepared baking sheet. Bake for 20-25 minutes, or until golden and crispy.

Meanwhile, brush the salmon fillets with olive oil and season with salt and pepper.

- Heat a grill pan or outdoor grill over medium-high heat. Grill the salmon for 3-4 minutes per side, or until cooked through.

- Arrange the asparagus on a baking sheet and drizzle with olive oil. Season with salt and pepper.
- Roast the asparagus in the oven for 10-15 minutes, or until tender and lightly browned.

Serve the grilled salmon with the roasted asparagus and sweet potato fries, topped with lemon wedges and chopped parsley.

Vegetable frittata with mixed greens salad

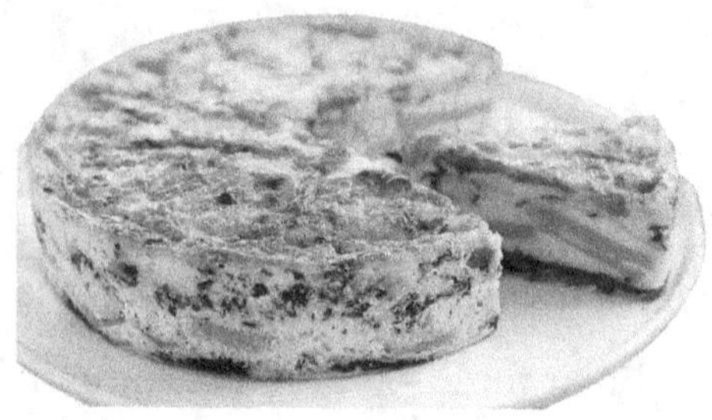

Ingredients:

8 large eggs

1/4 cup milk

Salt and pepper to taste

1 tablespoon olive oil

1/2 onion, chopped

1 bell pepper, chopped

1 zucchini, chopped

1 cup chopped kale

1/4 cup grated Parmesan cheese

4 cups mixed greens

1/2 cup cherry tomatoes, halved

1/4 cup sliced red onion

2 tablespoons balsamic vinegar

1 tablespoon olive oil

Salt and pepper to taste

Instructions:

- Preheat the oven to 375°F (190°C).
- In a large bowl, whisk together the eggs, milk, salt, and pepper until well combined.
- Heat the olive oil in a large oven-safe skillet over medium heat. Add the onion, bell pepper, and zucchini and cook for 5-7 minutes, or until the vegetables are tender.
- Stir in the chopped kale and cook for an additional 1-2 minutes, or until wilted.

- Pour the egg mixture into the skillet and sprinkle with Parmesan cheese. Cook for 2-3 minutes, or until the edges begin to set.
- Transfer the skillet to the preheated oven and bake for 10-12 minutes, or until the frittata is set and golden brown.

Meanwhile, in a large bowl, toss together the mixed greens, cherry tomatoes, and sliced red onion.

- In a small bowl, whisk together the balsamic vinegar, olive oil, salt, and pepper to make the dressing.

Serve the vegetable frittata with the mixed greens salad, topped with the balsamic vinaigrette.

Spaghetti squash with turkey meatballs and tomato sauce

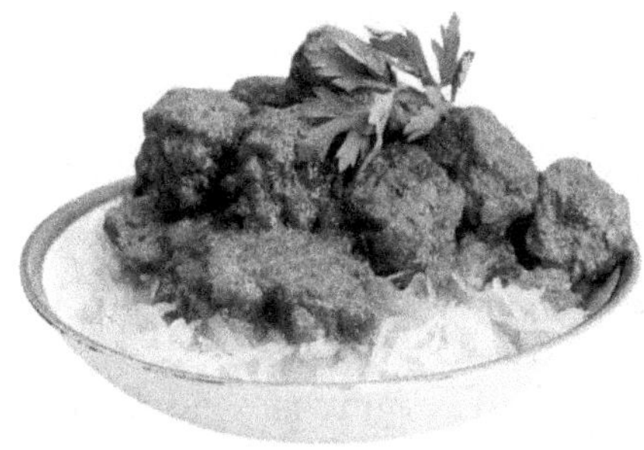

Ingredients:

1 spaghetti squash

1 pound ground turkey

1/4 cup almond flour

1 egg

1/4 cup grated Parmesan cheese

1/4 cup chopped fresh parsley

1 teaspoon dried oregano

1 teaspoon garlic powder

Salt and pepper to taste

1 tablespoon olive oil

1/2 onion, chopped

2 cloves garlic, minced

1 can (28 ounces) crushed tomatoes

1 teaspoon dried basil

1 teaspoon dried oregano

Salt and pepper to taste

Instructions:

- Preheat the oven to 375°F (190°C).
- Cut the spaghetti squash in half lengthwise and remove the seeds. Place the halves cut-side down on a baking sheet and bake for 35-40 minutes, or until the squash is tender.

While the squash is cooking, prepare the turkey meatballs.

- In a large bowl, combine the ground turkey, almond flour, egg, Parmesan cheese, parsley, oregano, garlic powder, salt, and pepper. Mix well and form into 1-inch balls.
- Heat the olive oil in a large skillet over medium heat. Add the onion and garlic and cook for 2-3 minutes, or until the onion is tender.
- Add the meatballs to the skillet and cook for 6-8 minutes, or until browned on all sides.

- Stir in the crushed tomatoes, basil, oregano, salt, and pepper. Bring to a simmer and cook for 10-15 minutes, or until the meatballs are cooked through and the sauce has thickened.
- Once the spaghetti squash is done, use a fork to scrape the flesh into spaghetti-like strands.

Serve the spaghetti squash topped with the turkey meatballs and tomato sauce.

Baked cod with roasted Brussels sprouts and sweet potato mash

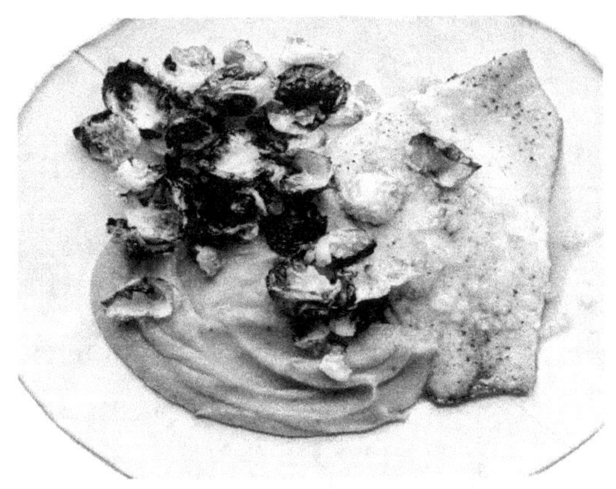

Ingredients:

4 cod fillets (4-6 ounces each)

1 tablespoon olive oil

1/2 teaspoon garlic powder

Salt and pepper to taste

1 pound Brussels sprouts, trimmed and halved

1 tablespoon balsamic vinegar

2 tablespoons olive oil

1 teaspoon dried thyme

Salt and pepper to taste

2 large sweet potatoes, peeled and cubed

1/4 cup milk

1 tablespoon butter

Salt and pepper to taste

Instructions:

- Preheat the oven to 400°F (200°C).
- Place the cod fillets on a baking sheet lined with parchment paper. Drizzle with olive oil and sprinkle with garlic powder, salt, and pepper. Bake for 12-15 minutes, or until the cod is cooked through and flakes easily with a fork.
- While the cod is cooking, prepare the Brussels sprouts. In a bowl, toss the Brussels sprouts with balsamic

vinegar, olive oil, thyme, salt, and pepper. Spread the Brussels sprouts out on a baking sheet and roast in the oven for 20-25 minutes, or until tender and lightly browned.

- While the Brussels sprouts are cooking, prepare the sweet potato mash. Boil the sweet potato cubes in a large pot of salted water for 15-20 minutes, or until tender. Drain and return the sweet potatoes to the pot.
- Add the milk and butter and mash until smooth. Season with salt and pepper to taste.

Serve the baked cod with the roasted Brussels sprouts and sweet potato mash.

Turkey and vegetable soup with whole-grain bread

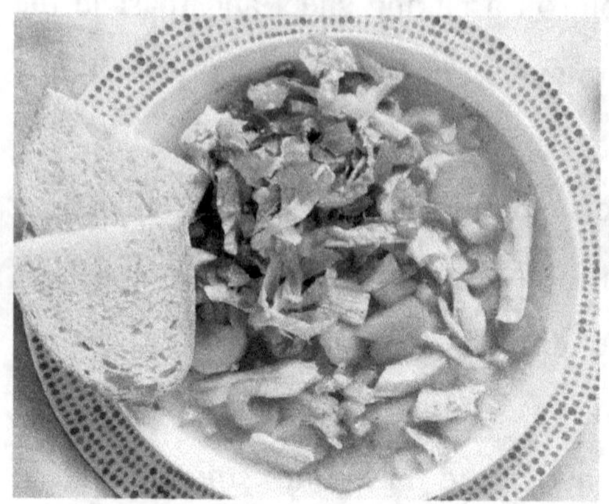

Ingredients:

1 tablespoon olive oil

1 onion, diced

2 cloves garlic, minced

2 carrots, peeled and diced

2 celery stalks, diced

1 red bell pepper, diced

1 zucchini, diced

4 cups low-sodium chicken or turkey broth

2 cups water

1 can (14.5 oz) diced tomatoes

1 teaspoon dried thyme

1/2 teaspoon dried rosemary

1/2 teaspoon dried oregano

Salt and pepper to taste

2 cups shredded cooked turkey

2 cups chopped kale or spinach

4 slices whole grain bread

Instructions:

- Heat the olive oil in a large pot over medium heat. Add the onion and garlic and sauté for 2-3 minutes, or until the onion is translucent.

- Add the carrots, celery, red bell pepper, and zucchini to the pot and sauté for another 5-7 minutes, or until the vegetables start to soften.

- Add the chicken or turkey broth, water, diced tomatoes, dried thyme, dried rosemary, dried oregano, salt, and pepper to the pot. Bring to a simmer and let cook for 10-15 minutes.

- Add the shredded turkey and chopped kale or spinach to the pot and simmer for another 5-7 minutes, or until the greens are wilted and the turkey is heated through.

Serve the soup hot with slices of whole-grain bread.

Grilled chicken Caesar salad

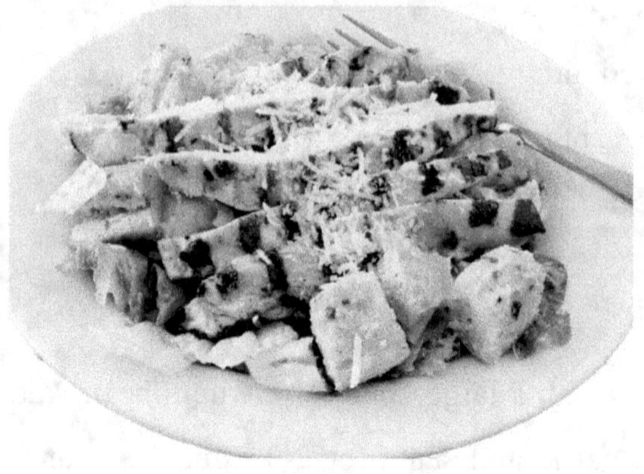

Ingredients:

2 chicken breasts

Salt and pepper

Olive oil

1 head of romaine lettuce, chopped

1/2 cup croutons

1/4 cup grated parmesan cheese

Caesar dressing (store-bought or homemade)

Lemon wedges, for serving

Instructions:

- Preheat a grill or grill pan to medium-high heat.
- Season the chicken breasts with salt and pepper and drizzle with olive oil.

- Grill the chicken breasts for 6-8 minutes per side, or until fully cooked. Set aside to cool.
- In a large bowl, toss the chopped romaine lettuce with croutons, grated parmesan cheese, and Caesar dressing.
- Slice the grilled chicken breasts and add to the salad.
- Toss the salad to coat with dressing.

Serve with lemon wedges on the side.

Lentil and vegetable curry with brown rice

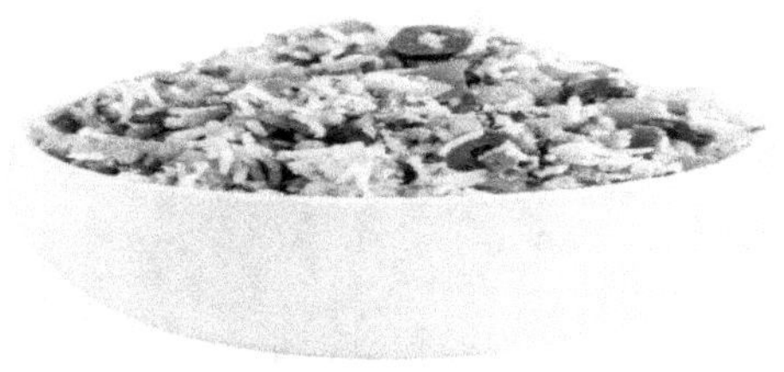

Ingredients:

1 cup brown rice

2 cups water

1 tablespoon olive oil

1 onion, chopped

2 cloves garlic, minced

1 tablespoon curry powder

1 teaspoon ground cumin

1 teaspoon ground coriander

1/2 teaspoon ground turmeric

1/4 teaspoon cayenne pepper

2 cups vegetable broth

1 can (14.5 oz) diced tomatoes

1 can (15 oz) lentils, rinsed and drained

1 cup chopped carrots

1 cup chopped bell peppers

1 cup chopped zucchini

Salt and pepper to taste

Chopped cilantro for garnish (optional)

Instructions:

- In a medium saucepan, bring the water to a boil. Add the brown rice, reduce heat to low, and simmer for 40-45 minutes or until tender.

- In a large skillet or saucepan, heat the olive oil over medium-high heat.

- Add the onion and garlic and sauté until soft and translucent.
- Add the curry powder, cumin, coriander, turmeric, and cayenne pepper and stir to combine.
- Add the vegetable broth, diced tomatoes, lentils, carrots, bell peppers, and zucchini. Stir to combine.
- Bring the mixture to a boil, then reduce heat to low and simmer for 20-25 minutes or until the vegetables are tender.
- Season with salt and pepper to taste.

Serve the curry over brown rice, and garnish with chopped cilantro if desired.

Grilled chicken skewers with mixed vegetables and brown rice

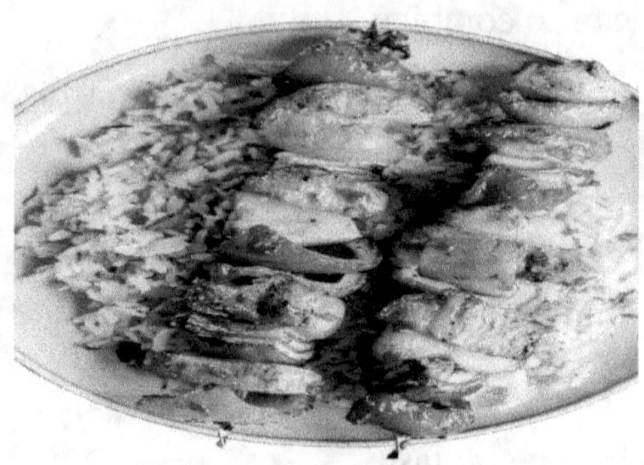

Ingredients:

1 lb boneless, skinless chicken breast, cut into 1-inch cubes

2 tablespoons olive oil

2 tablespoons fresh lemon juice

1 teaspoon dried oregano

1/2 teaspoon garlic powder

Salt and pepper to taste

1 red bell pepper, seeded and cut into 1-inch pieces

1 yellow bell pepper, seeded and cut into 1-inch pieces

1 red onion, cut into 1-inch pieces

8-10 cherry tomatoes

1 cup uncooked brown rice

2 cups water or chicken broth

Chopped fresh parsley for garnish (optional)

Instructions:

- In a bowl, whisk together the olive oil, lemon juice, oregano, garlic powder, salt, and pepper. Add the chicken and toss to coat. Marinate in the refrigerator for at least 30 minutes, up to 2 hours.
- Preheat the grill to medium-high heat.
- Thread the marinated chicken, bell peppers, red onion, and cherry tomatoes onto skewers.
- Grill the skewers for 10-12 minutes, flipping once, until the chicken is cooked through and the vegetables are tender.
- While the skewers are grilling, prepare the brown rice. In a medium saucepan, bring the water or chicken broth to a boil. Add the brown rice and stir to combine. Reduce the heat to low, cover, and simmer for 40-45 minutes or until the rice is tender and the liquid is absorbed.

Serve the grilled chicken skewers and mixed vegetables over brown rice, and garnish with chopped fresh parsley.

Grilled salmon with mixed vegetables and brown rice

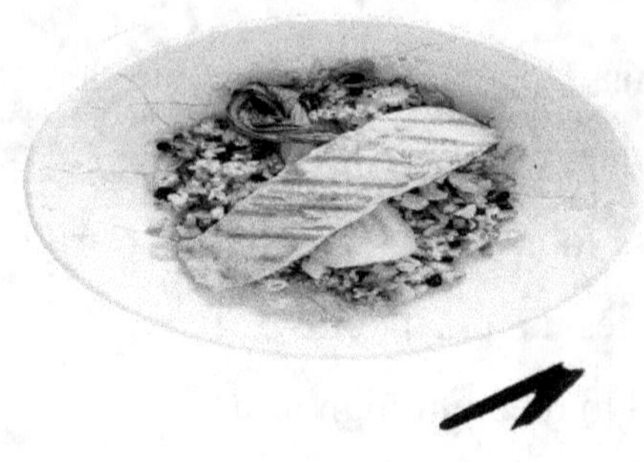

Ingredients:

4 salmon fillets

1 red bell pepper, sliced

1 yellow bell pepper, sliced

1 small zucchini, sliced

1 small yellow squash, sliced

1 small red onion, sliced

2 cloves garlic, minced

2 tablespoons olive oil

1 teaspoon dried thyme

Salt and pepper, to taste

2 cups cooked brown rice

Instructions:

- Preheat the grill to medium-high heat.
- In a large bowl, mix together the sliced bell peppers, zucchini, yellow squash, red onion, minced garlic, olive oil, dried thyme, salt, and pepper until the vegetables are coated in the oil and seasoning.
- Thread the vegetables onto skewers, alternating the different vegetables.
- Brush the salmon fillets with olive oil and season with salt and pepper.
- Place the vegetable skewers and salmon fillets onto the preheated grill.
- Grill the vegetables for 8-10 minutes, turning occasionally, until they are charred and tender.
- Grill the salmon for 4-6 minutes per side, or until the salmon flakes easily with a fork.

Serve the grilled salmon with mixed vegetables and brown rice.

Greek salad with grilled chicken or tofu

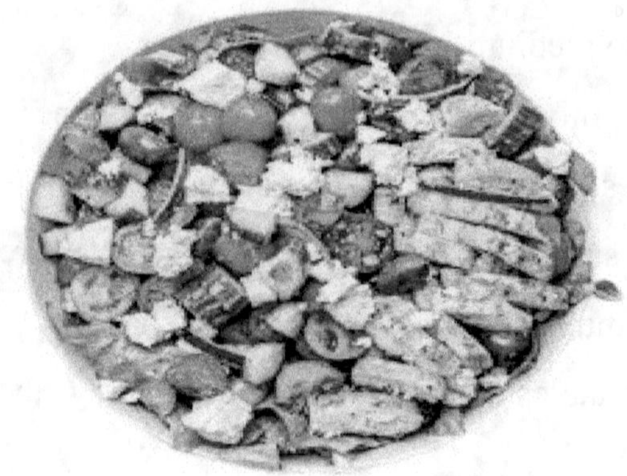

Ingredients:

4 cups mixed greens

1/2 red onion, sliced

1/2 cucumber, sliced

1/2 red bell pepper, sliced

1/2 yellow bell pepper, sliced

1/2 cup cherry tomatoes, halved

1/2 cup kalamata olives, pitted

1/2 cup crumbled feta cheese

2 chicken breasts or 1 block of tofu

2 tablespoons olive oil

1 tablespoon lemon juice

1 teaspoon dried oregano

Salt and pepper, to taste

Instructions:

- Preheat a grill or grill pan to medium-high heat.
- In a large bowl, combine the mixed greens, sliced red onion, cucumber, red bell pepper, yellow bell pepper, cherry tomatoes, and kalamata olives.
- In a separate bowl, whisk together the olive oil, lemon juice, dried oregano, salt, and pepper.
- If using chicken, season with salt and pepper and grill for 6-8 minutes per side, or until cooked through. If using tofu, slice into 1/2-inch thick pieces, brush with olive oil and grill for 3-4 minutes per side.
- Once cooked, remove the chicken or tofu from the grill and let it rest for a few minutes before slicing.
- Add the sliced chicken or tofu to the salad and drizzle with the dressing.

Top with crumbled feta cheese and serve.

Grilled chicken with roasted zucchini and tomato sauce

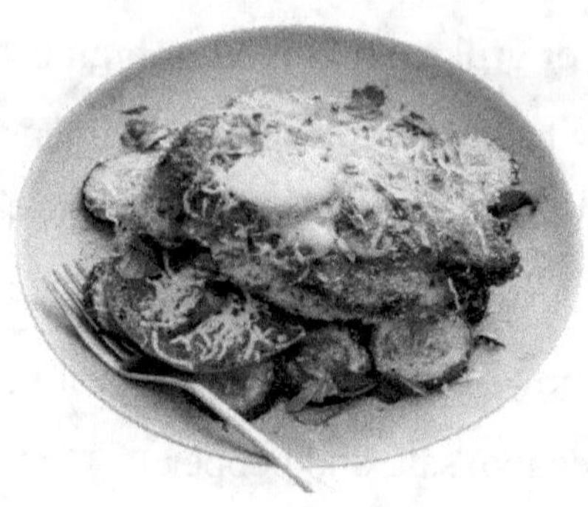

Ingredients:

4 boneless, skinless chicken breasts

2 large zucchinis, sliced into rounds

2 cups of tomato sauce (store-bought or homemade)

2 tbsp olive oil

1 tsp dried oregano

1/2 tsp garlic powder

Salt and pepper, to taste

Instructions:

- Preheat your grill to medium-high heat.

- Brush both sides of the chicken breasts with olive oil, and season with oregano, garlic powder, salt, and pepper.
- Grill the chicken for about 6-8 minutes per side, or until the internal temperature reaches 165°F.
- While the chicken is cooking, toss the sliced zucchini with 1 tbsp of olive oil, salt, and pepper, and spread them out in a single layer on a baking sheet.
- Roast the zucchini in the oven at 400°F for about 15-20 minutes, or until tender and slightly browned.
- In a small saucepan, heat the tomato sauce until it's warm.

Serve the grilled chicken with the roasted zucchini and tomato sauce on top.

Baked sweet potato with black beans and avocado

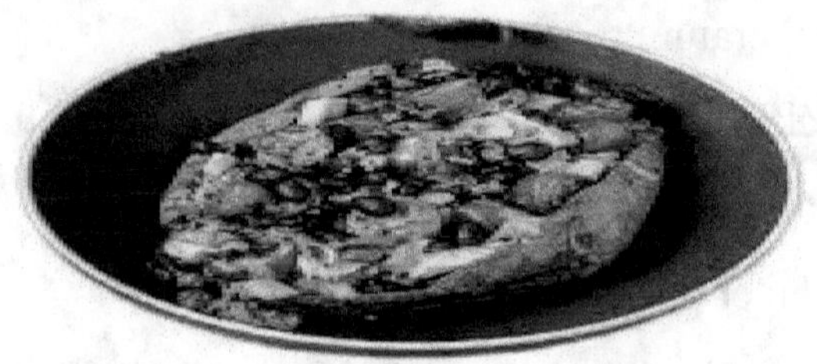

Ingredients:

4 medium-sized sweet potatoes

1 can (15 oz) black beans, drained and rinsed

1 avocado, diced

1/2 red onion, diced

1 jalapeño pepper, seeded and minced

1 lime, juiced

2 tbsp chopped cilantro

1 tbsp olive oil

1/2 tsp ground cumin

Salt and pepper, to taste

Instructions:

- Preheat your oven to 400°F.

- Wash and dry the sweet potatoes, then prick them all over with a fork.

- Place the sweet potatoes on a baking sheet and bake for 45-50 minutes, or until tender.

- While the sweet potatoes are baking, prepare the black bean and avocado topping. In a mixing bowl, combine the black beans, diced avocado, red onion, minced jalapeño, lime juice, cilantro, olive oil, cumin, salt, and pepper. Mix well.

- When the sweet potatoes are done, remove them from the oven and let them cool for a few minutes.

- Cut a slit down the middle of each sweet potato and fluff up the insides with a fork.

- Top each sweet potato with the black bean and avocado mixture.

Serve hot and enjoy!

Grilled shrimp and vegetable skewers with brown rice

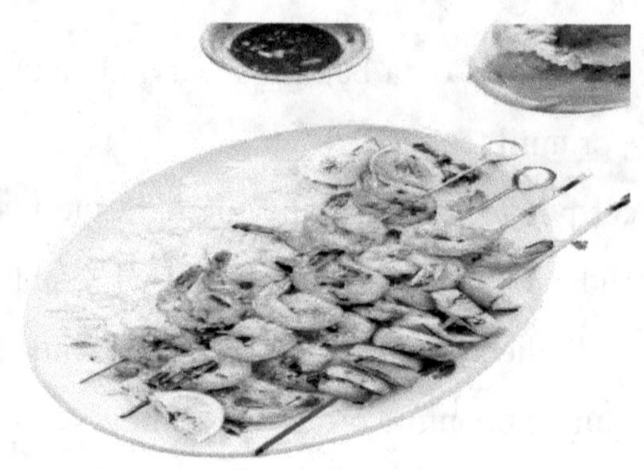

Ingredients:

1 lb shrimp, peeled and deveined

1 red bell pepper, cut into chunks

1 yellow bell pepper, cut into chunks

1 red onion, cut into chunks

1 zucchini, sliced

2 cloves garlic, minced

2 tbsp olive oil

1 tsp paprika

1/2 tsp ground cumin

Salt and pepper to taste

1 cup brown rice, cooked

Instructions:

- In a bowl, combine the shrimp, bell peppers, red onion, zucchini, garlic, olive oil, paprika, cumin, salt, and pepper. Toss to coat everything well.
- Thread the shrimp and vegetables onto skewers, alternating between shrimp and vegetables.
- Heat a grill or grill pan over medium-high heat. Once hot, add the skewers and grill for 2-3 minutes per side or until the shrimp are pink and cooked through.

Serve the shrimp and vegetable skewers with cooked brown rice.

Spinach and mushroom omelet with whole-grain toast

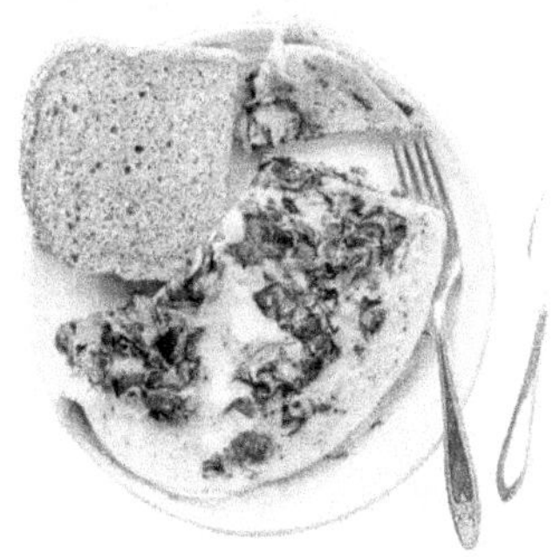

Ingredients:

3 eggs

1/4 cup milk

1 cup fresh spinach leaves

1/2 cup sliced mushrooms

1/4 cup diced onion

1 clove garlic, minced

1 tbsp olive oil

Salt and pepper to taste

2 slices of whole-grain bread

Instructions:

- In a bowl, whisk together the eggs, milk, salt, and pepper until well combined.
- Heat the olive oil in a nonstick skillet over medium heat. Once hot, add the onion and garlic and sauté until the onion is translucent.
- Add the mushrooms and cook until they release their liquid and begin to brown about 5 minutes.
- Add the spinach to the skillet and cook until wilted, about 1-2 minutes.

- Pour the egg mixture over the vegetables in the skillet and cook until the bottom is set, about 2-3 minutes.
- Use a spatula to fold the omelet in half and cook for an additional 1-2 minutes or until the eggs are fully cooked.
- Toast the slices of whole grain bread.

Serve the omelet with the toast on the side.

Broiled tilapia with mixed vegetables and brown rice

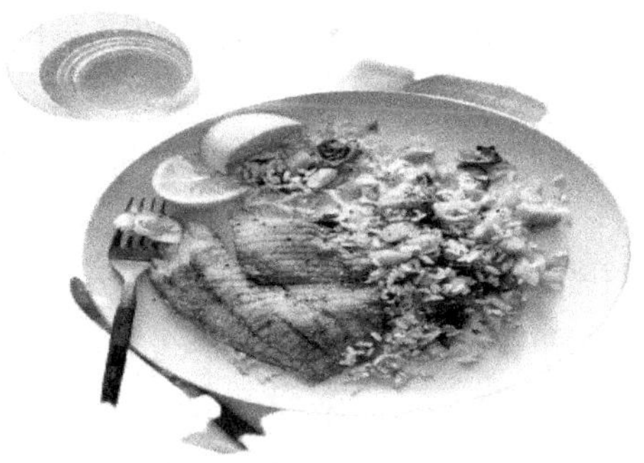

Ingredients:

4 tilapia fillets

2 cups of mixed vegetables (carrots, bell peppers, onions, zucchini, etc.)

1 cup of brown rice

2 tablespoons of olive oil

2 cloves of garlic, minced

Salt and pepper to taste

Lemon wedges for garnish

Instructions:

- Preheat the broiler in your oven.
- Cook the brown rice according to the package instructions.
- Cut the mixed vegetables into bite-sized pieces.
- Heat one tablespoon of olive oil in a large skillet over medium heat. Add the minced garlic and cook until fragrant, about 1 minute.
- Add the mixed vegetables to the skillet and sauté until they are tender, about 8-10 minutes. Season with salt and pepper to taste.
- Brush the tilapia fillets with the remaining tablespoon of olive oil and season with salt and pepper.
- Place the tilapia fillets on a baking sheet and broil for 6-8 minutes, or until cooked through.

Serve the broiled tilapia with sautéed vegetables and brown rice.
Garnish with lemon wedges, if desired.

Vegetable and lentil shepherd's pie

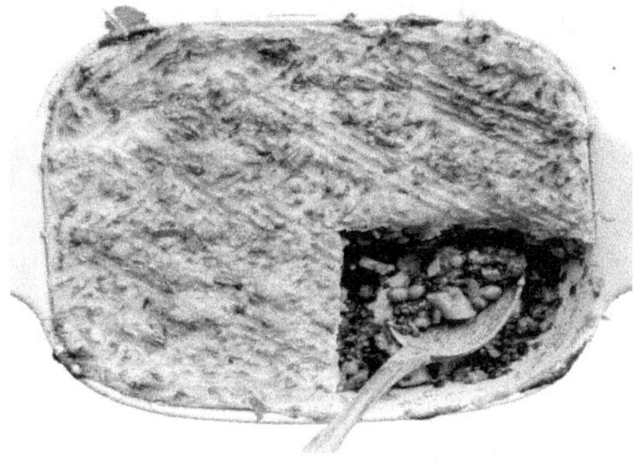

Ingredients:

1 tablespoon olive oil

1 onion, diced

2 carrots, peeled and diced

2 stalks celery, diced

3 cloves garlic, minced

1 teaspoon dried thyme

1 teaspoon dried rosemary

1 teaspoon paprika

1 teaspoon salt

1/2 teaspoon black pepper

1 cup green or brown lentils, rinsed and drained

1 1/2 cups vegetable broth

1 tablespoon tomato paste

1 bay leaf

2 large sweet potatoes, peeled and cubed

2 tablespoons butter

1/4 cup milk

Salt and pepper to taste

Instructions:

- Preheat the oven to 375°F (190°C).
- In a large skillet, heat the olive oil over medium heat. Add the onion, carrots, celery, and garlic, and sauté until the vegetables are tender, about 10 minutes.
- Add the dried thyme, dried rosemary, paprika, salt, and black pepper, and stir well to combine.
- Add the lentils, vegetable broth, tomato paste, and bay leaf, and stir to combine. Bring the mixture to a boil, then reduce the heat to low and let it simmer for 20-25 minutes until the lentils are tender and the liquid has been absorbed.

- While the lentils are cooking, boil the sweet potatoes in a separate pot of salted water until they are fork-tender. Drain them and mash them with the butter and milk until smooth. Season with salt and pepper to taste.
- Remove the bay leaf from the lentil mixture and transfer it to a large baking dish. Spread the mashed sweet potatoes over the top of the lentils.
- Bake the shepherd's pie in the preheated oven for 20-25 minutes, until the top is golden brown and the filling is bubbling.

Serve hot.

Grilled chicken and vegetable kebab with quinoa

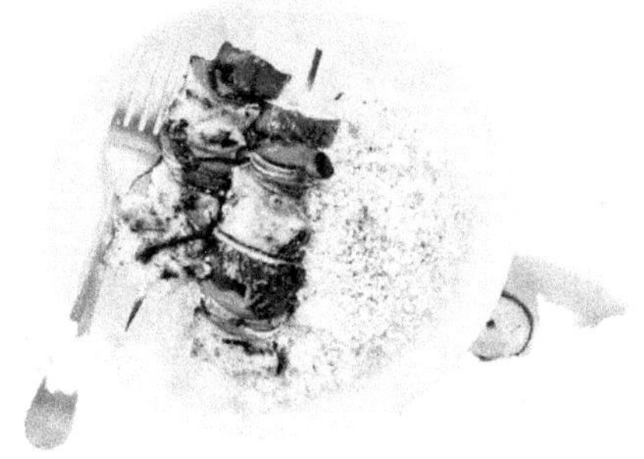

Ingredients:

1 pound boneless, skinless chicken breast, cut into 1-inch cubes

2 bell peppers, seeded and cut into 1-inch pieces

1 zucchini, cut into 1-inch pieces

1 onion, cut into 1-inch pieces

8-10 wooden skewers

1 tablespoon olive oil

1 teaspoon dried oregano

1 teaspoon dried basil

Salt and pepper to taste

1 cup quinoa

2 cups water

1 tablespoon olive oil

Instructions:

- Soak the wooden skewers in water for at least 30 minutes to prevent burning.
- Preheat the grill to medium-high heat.
- In a large bowl, combine the chicken, peppers, zucchini, onion, olive oil, oregano, basil, salt, and pepper. Toss to coat the vegetables and chicken evenly.

- Thread the chicken and vegetables onto the skewers, alternating the pieces.
- Grill the skewers for 10-12 minutes, turning occasionally, until the chicken is cooked through and the vegetables are tender and slightly charred.
- While the skewers are grilling, prepare the quinoa. Rinse the quinoa in a fine-mesh strainer and transfer it to a medium saucepan.
- Add 2 cups of water and bring to a boil over high heat. Reduce the heat to low, cover, and simmer for 15-20 minutes, or until the quinoa is tender and the water is absorbed. Fluff with a fork.
- Drizzle the cooked quinoa with olive oil and season with salt and pepper to taste.

Serve the grilled chicken and vegetable kebabs with the quinoa on the side.

Grilled steak with roasted sweet potato and green beans

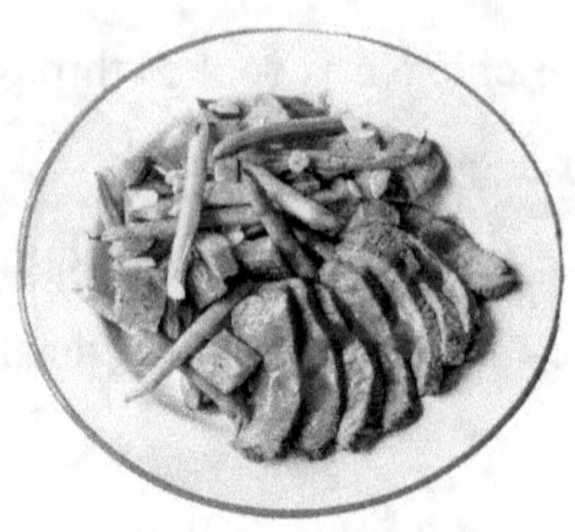

Ingredients:

1 pound sirloin steak

2 medium sweet potatoes, peeled and chopped

1 pound green beans, trimmed

2 tablespoons olive oil

Salt and pepper to taste

Instructions:

- Preheat your grill to medium-high heat.
- Rub the steak with olive oil, salt, and pepper.

- Place the steak on the grill and cook for 4-5 minutes per side for medium-rare, or until it reaches your desired doneness.

- While the steak is cooking, toss the chopped sweet potatoes and green beans in a bowl with olive oil, salt, and pepper.

- Spread the vegetables out on a baking sheet and roast in the oven at 400°F for 20-25 minutes, or until the sweet potatoes are tender and the green beans are slightly charred.

Slice the steak against the grain and serve with the roasted sweet potatoes and green beans.

Grilled portobello mushrooms with mixed greens and balsamic vinaigrette

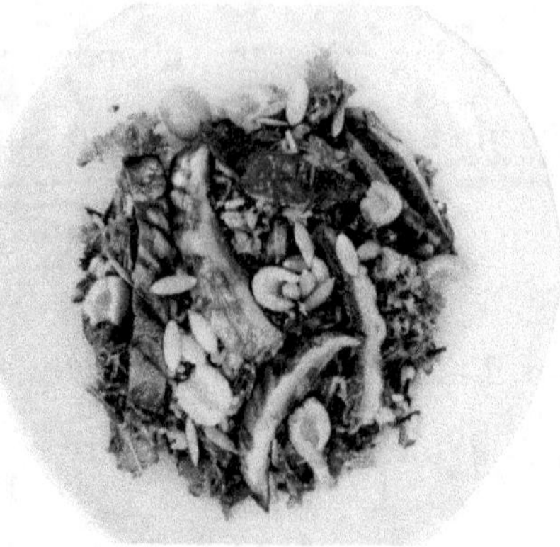

Ingredients:

4 large portobello mushroom caps

2 cloves garlic, minced

2 tablespoons balsamic vinegar

2 tablespoons olive oil

1 teaspoon Dijon mustard

Salt and pepper to taste

6 cups mixed greens

1/4 cup chopped walnuts

1/4 cup crumbled feta cheese

Instructions:

- Preheat the grill to medium-high heat.
- In a small bowl, whisk together garlic, balsamic vinegar, olive oil, Dijon mustard, salt, and pepper.
- Brush the portobello mushrooms with the balsamic mixture and place them on the grill, gill-side down. Grill for 4-5 minutes per side, or until they are tender.
- In a large bowl, toss together the mixed greens, chopped walnuts, and crumbled feta cheese.

Serve the grilled portobello mushrooms over the mixed greens salad. Drizzle any remaining balsamic mixture over the top.

Turkey chili with mixed vegetables and quinoa

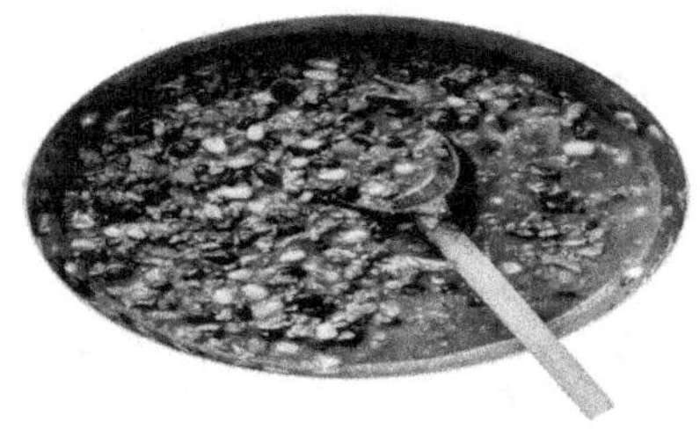

Ingredients:

1 pound ground turkey

1 can (15 oz) black beans, drained and rinsed

1 can (15 oz) kidney beans, drained and rinsed

1 can (15 oz) diced tomatoes

1 green bell pepper, diced

1 red bell pepper, diced

1 onion, diced

1 jalapeño pepper, seeded and diced

2 cloves garlic, minced

1 tablespoon chili powder

1 teaspoon cumin

1 teaspoon paprika

1 teaspoon oregano

1/2 teaspoon salt

1/4 teaspoon black pepper

3 cups low-sodium chicken broth

1 cup uncooked quinoa

1 tablespoon olive oil

Instructions:

- Preheat a large pot over medium heat. Add the olive oil and ground turkey. Cook for 5-7 minutes until the turkey is browned and cooked through.
- Add the diced onion, green bell pepper, red bell pepper, jalapeño pepper, and minced garlic. Stir to combine and cook for an additional 3-5 minutes until the vegetables are slightly softened.
- Add the chili powder, cumin, paprika, oregano, salt, and black pepper. Stir to combine and cook for an additional 2-3 minutes until the spices are fragrant.
- Add the black beans, kidney beans, diced tomatoes, and chicken broth. Bring to a simmer and let cook for 10-15 minutes.
- Add the quinoa to the pot and stir to combine. Let the chili simmer for an additional 15-20 minutes, or until the quinoa is cooked through and the chili has thickened.

Serve hot and enjoy!

CHAPTER 4

SUBSTITUTION AND TECHNIQUES

Ingredients substitution

Modifying recipes to fit individual dietary needs can seem overwhelming at first, but it's actually quite simple. Here are some tips for modifying recipes:

Identify the ingredients that need to be modified: Take a look at the recipe and identify the ingredients that need to be modified to fit your dietary needs. For example, if you're following a low-sodium diet, you may need to reduce or eliminate added salt.

Swap ingredients: Consider swapping out ingredients that don't fit your dietary needs with ones that do. For example, if you're following a vegan diet, you can substitute plant-based milk for cow's milk in a recipe.

Adjust cooking times and temperatures: Some modifications may require adjustments to cooking times and temperatures. For example, if you're using a sugar substitute in a baking recipe, you may need to reduce the cooking time and temperature to prevent the recipe from burning.

Experiment with flavor: Modifying recipes can be an opportunity to experiment with different flavors and spices. For example, if you're following a low-sodium diet, you can experiment with using different herbs and spices to add flavor to your meals.

By following these tips, you can modify recipes to fit your individual dietary needs without sacrificing flavor or nutrition.

Food substitutions can be helpful when modifying recipes to fit dietary needs or preferences. Here are some common food substitutions:

Milk: You can substitute cow's milk with plant-based milk like almond, soy, or oat milk.

Butter: You can substitute butter with olive oil, coconut oil, or avocado oil.

Eggs: You can substitute eggs with applesauce, mashed banana, or a commercial egg substitute.

Flour: You can substitute all-purpose flour with whole wheat flour, almond flour, or coconut flour.

Sugar: You can substitute granulated sugar with honey, maple syrup, or stevia.

Salt: You can substitute salt with herbs and spices like garlic, cumin, or paprika.

Meat: You can substitute meat with plant-based protein like tofu, tempeh, or legumes.

It's important to note that substitutions can impact the flavor and texture of a recipe. Therefore, it's a good idea to experiment with different substitutions to find the one that works best for your recipe and taste preferences.

Healthy cooking techniques

Cooking techniques can significantly impact the nutritional content of your meals. Here are some cooking techniques that promote heart health:

Grilling or broiling: Grilling or broiling lean proteins like chicken, fish, or vegetables is a great way to reduce the amount of added fat in your meals. Just be sure to avoid charring your food as this can increase the formation of harmful compounds.

Steaming: Steaming is a great way to cook vegetables while preserving their nutrients. It also requires no added fat, making it a heart-healthy cooking method.

Stir-frying: Stir-frying is a quick and easy way to cook vegetables, lean proteins, and whole grains. Use a small amount of healthy oil like olive or avocado oil and add flavorful herbs and spices to boost the flavor.

Baking or roasting: Baking or roasting is a healthy cooking method that requires little to no added fat. This method is especially great for cooking heart-healthy vegetables like sweet potatoes, carrots, and Brussels sprouts.

Boiling: Boiling is a simple cooking method that can be used for cooking whole grains like brown rice or quinoa. It's important to keep an eye on the pot and avoid overcooking as this can lead to a loss of nutrients.

Poaching: Poaching is a gentle cooking method that involves cooking food in liquid like water or broth. This method is great for cooking delicate proteins like fish and chicken.

Using healthy fats: When cooking with oil, choose healthy fats like olive oil, avocado oil, or coconut oil. These oils are rich in heart-healthy monounsaturated and polyunsaturated fats.

CONCLUSION

In conclusion, healthy eating is crucial for maintaining good health and well-being, and this cookbook provides a wealth of information and resources to help you achieve your goals. By cooking your meals at home and using the tips for meal planning, grocery shopping, and food prep, you can make healthy eating a more manageable and enjoyable part of your daily routine. With a variety of healthy meal recipes and a focus on macronutrients and micronutrients, this cookbook provides everything you need to start cooking delicious and nutritious meals at home. Whether you are looking to lose weight, improve your energy levels, or simply feel better in your body, this cookbook is a valuable resource for anyone looking to adopt a healthier lifestyle.

ENCOURAGEMENT

Embarking on a healthy lifestyle journey is a significant step towards improving your overall well-being, and it's important to recognize the progress you've made so far. Remember that change takes time, and there will be ups and downs along the way. However, with dedication and consistency, you can achieve your health and wellness goals.

Don't be too hard on yourself if you slip up or make mistakes. Use these experiences as opportunities to learn and grow, and don't let them discourage you from continuing on your healthy lifestyle journey. Celebrate your successes, no matter how small they may seem, and keep pushing yourself towards your goals.

Surround yourself with supportive people who will encourage and motivate you along the way. Seek out resources and tools, like this cookbook, that can help you stay on track and make healthy eating more manageable and enjoyable.

Remember that healthy eating is just one component of a healthy lifestyle. Incorporating physical activity, stress management, and self-care practices into your daily routine can also help you achieve your health and wellness goals. Most importantly, be kind to yourself and trust the process. Your commitment to a healthy lifestyle will pay off in the long run, and you'll be amazed at the positive changes you'll see in your body, mind, and overall well-being.

MEAL PLANNER

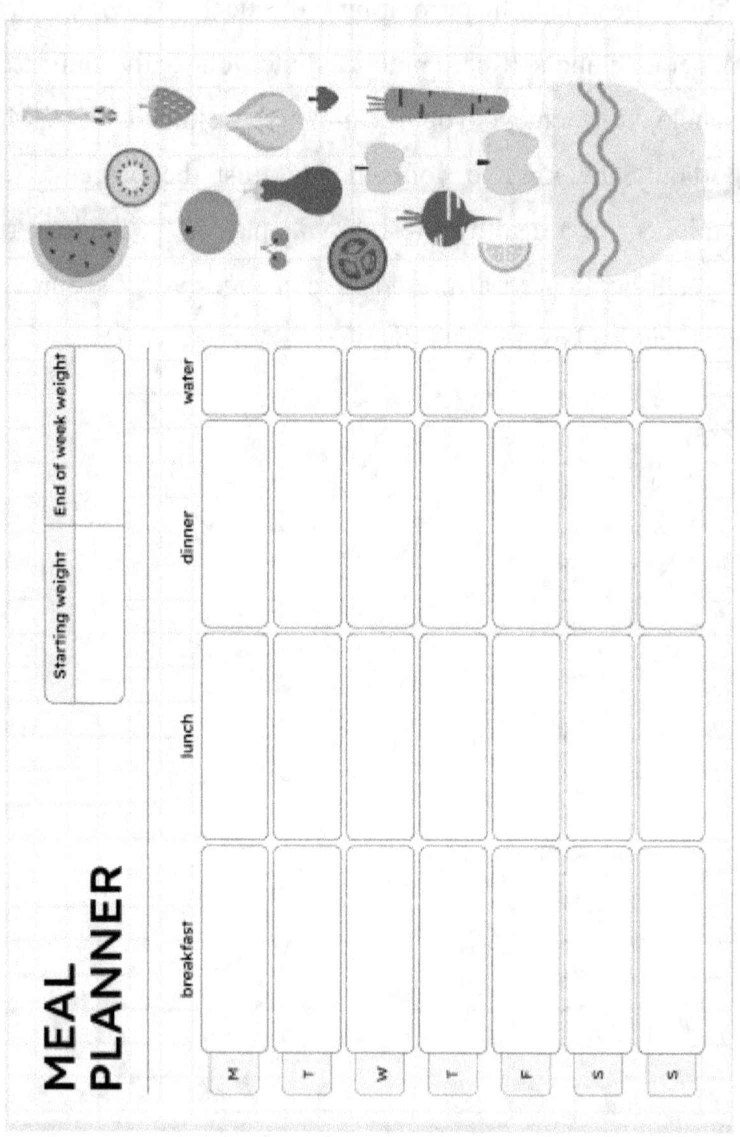

MEAL PLANNER

Starting weight	End of week weight

	breakfast	lunch	dinner	water
M				
T				
W				
T				
F				
S				
S				

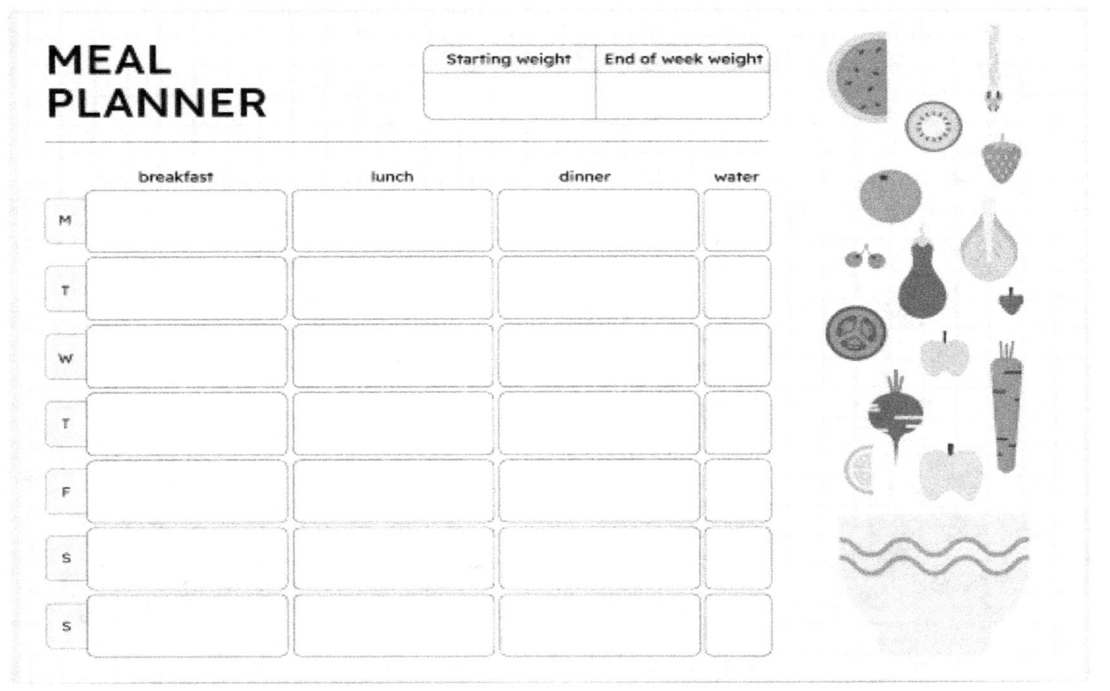

MEAL PLANNER

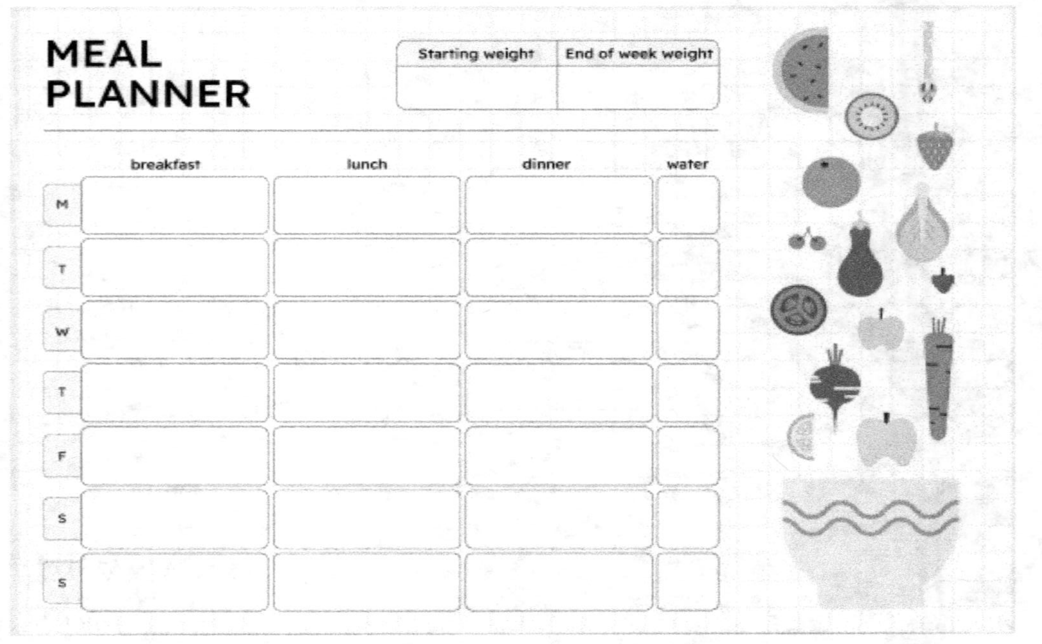

	Starting weight	End of week weight

	breakfast	lunch	dinner	water
M				
T				
W				
T				
F				
S				
S				

MEAL PLANNER

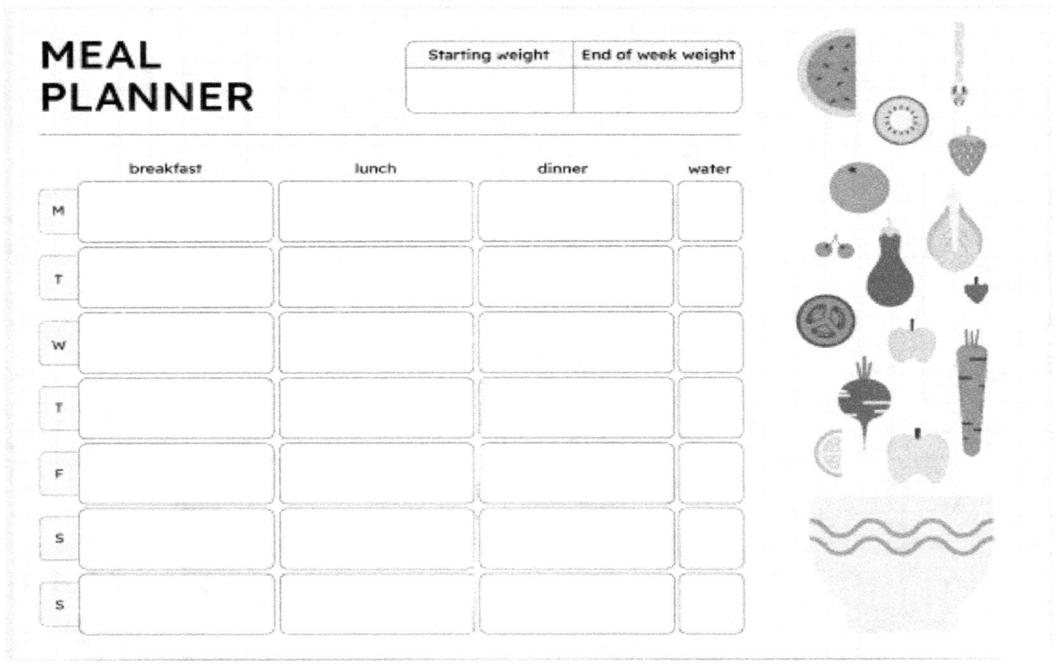

	Starting weight	End of week weight

	breakfast	lunch	dinner	water
M				
T				
W				
T				
F				
S				
S				

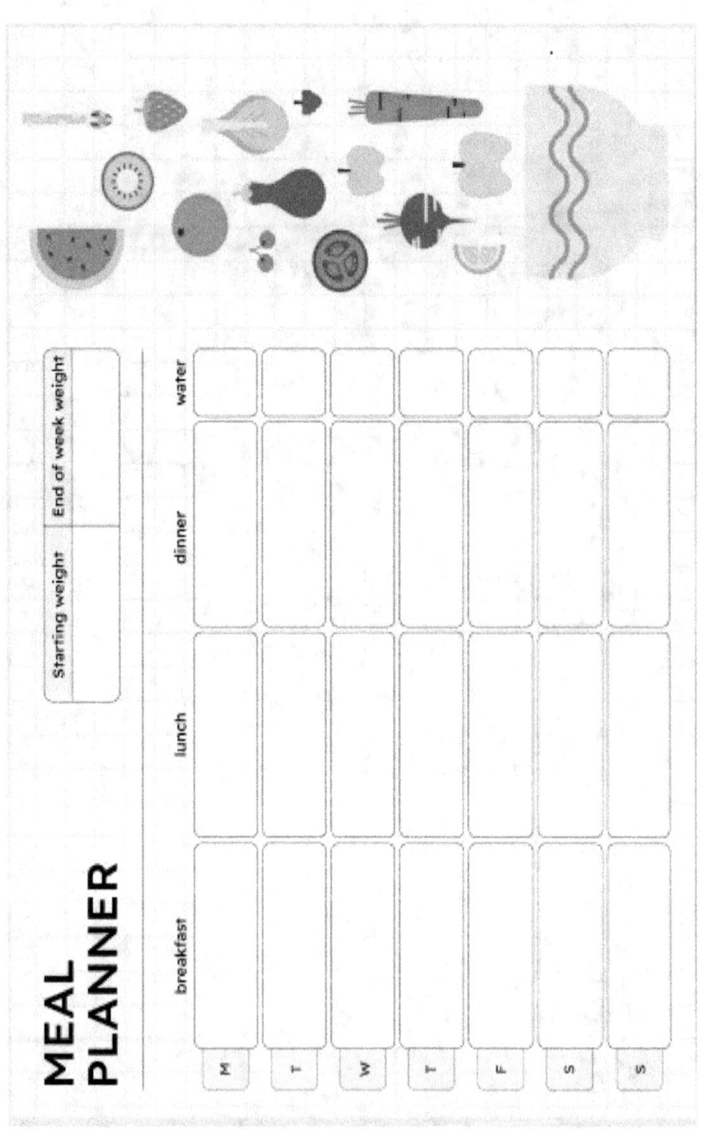

MEAL
PLANNER
Starting weight
End of week weight
breakfast
lunch
dinner
water
M
T
W
T
F
S
S